HEALTHY SLEEP

Understanding Sleep to Improve Your Health

Copyright Notice

Table of Contents

Introduction

Sleep, like nutrition and physical activity, is a critical determinant of health and well-being. Sleep is a basic requirement for infant, child, and adolescent health and development. Sleep loss and untreated sleep disorders influence basic patterns of behavior that negatively affect family health and interpersonal relationships. Fatigue and sleepiness can reduce productivity and increase the chance for mishaps such as medical errors and motor vehicle or industrial accidents.

Adequate sleep is necessary to:

- *Fight off infection*
- *Support the metabolism of sugar to prevent diabetes*
- *Perform well in school*
- *Work effectively and safely*

In Healthy Sleep we have tried to provide you with knowledge of how adequate sleep and treatment of sleep disorders improve health, productivity, wellness, quality of life, and safety on roads and in the workplace.

We hope you use this information to improve your life.

Sincerely,

R Healthy Living Solutions

Understanding Sleep

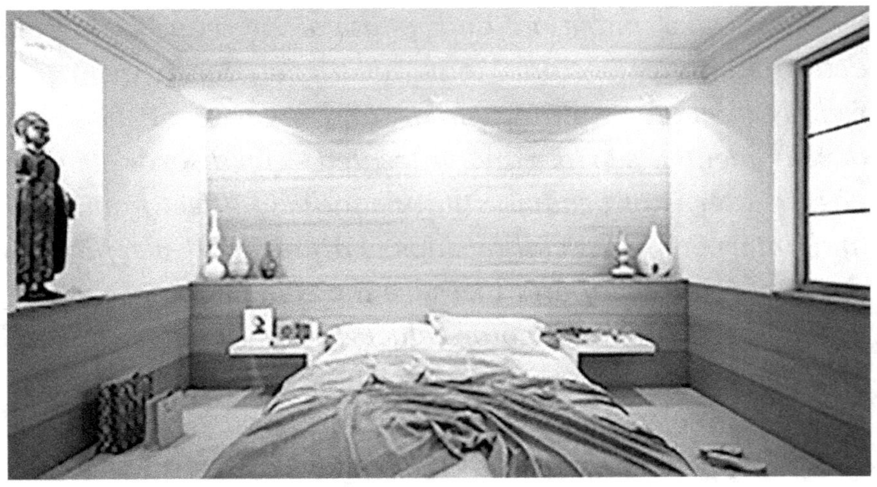

Sleep serves both a physical and psychological need that is required throughout your life. You know that sleep is important, and that you don't feel well when you don't get it. Unfortunately, in our fast-paced, modern world filled with technology, sleep is often the first thing we sacrifice.

After all, we all only get 24 hours each day. Why not try to fit as many things as possible into these 24 hours? Perhaps you have an important project that is due tomorrow. Well, you can always cut out a couple of hours of sleep to get it done, right?

Unfortunately, that is how more and more people are viewing sleep. They see it as an annoyance or an interruption to getting more things done in a day. Teenagers and adults are all suffering the negative consequences of this attitude towards sleep. Health suffers when sleep is put on the back burner.

However, some people are trying to prioritize sleep. They really want to get more sleep or want to sleep better, but they continue to wake up feeling unrefreshed. Perhaps, the stress in their lives is interfering with their sleep, or there are things that they need to change to get the sleep their bodies crave.

In any case, it is time to see sleep for what it really is - a necessary component to good health, both in the short-term and the long-term. Getting adequate, quality sleep is just as important as what you eat and how much you exercise. Not getting enough sleep is linked to numerous health concerns and diseases. Even serious diseases, such as cancer, have been linked to inadequate levels of sleep and disrupted sleep systems in people who work shifts.

Why we need sleep

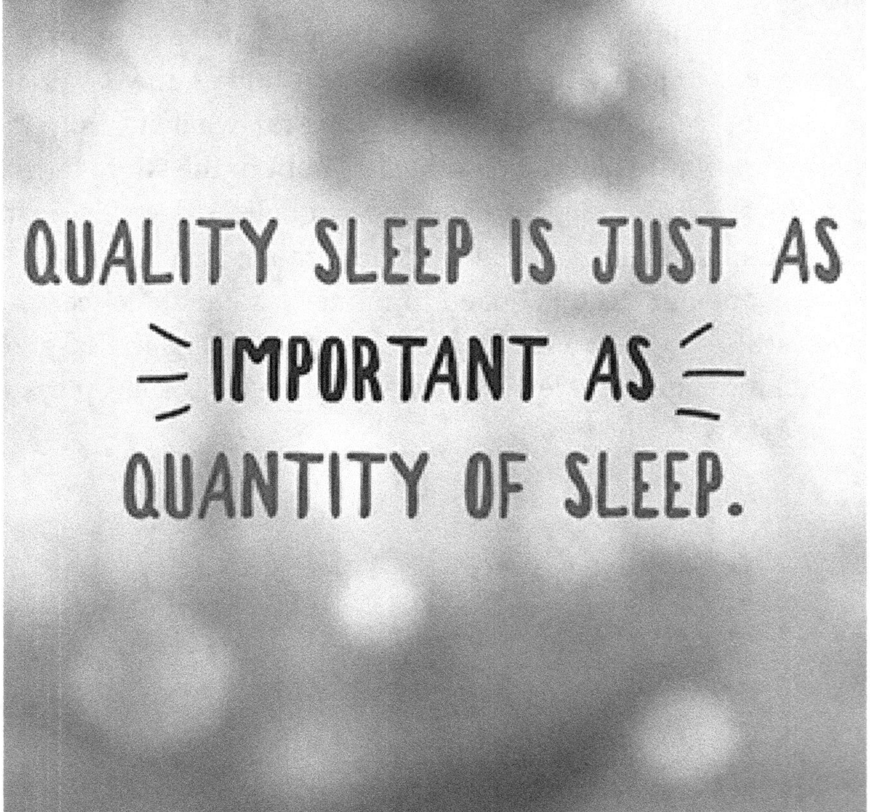

People may be wondering how losing out on sleep can cause all these health issues. The reason your body and mind can start to become affected by a lack sleep is because sleep is something we all need.

While we sleep our body is restoring and strengthening itself. With this being the case, it should be easy to understand why a person's body may seem to be failing when they have not slept because they do not have that much needed time to restore and strengthen.

Along with allowing people to restore and strengthen their bodies, sleep also allows people to consolidate their memories. This is when the information that is taken in during the day is processed and taken from short-term memory to long-term memory.

Therefore, memory can be affected when a person does not sleep. There is less time for them to process thoughts and memories and place them in their long-term memory where they should be.

Understanding the Different Stages of Sleep

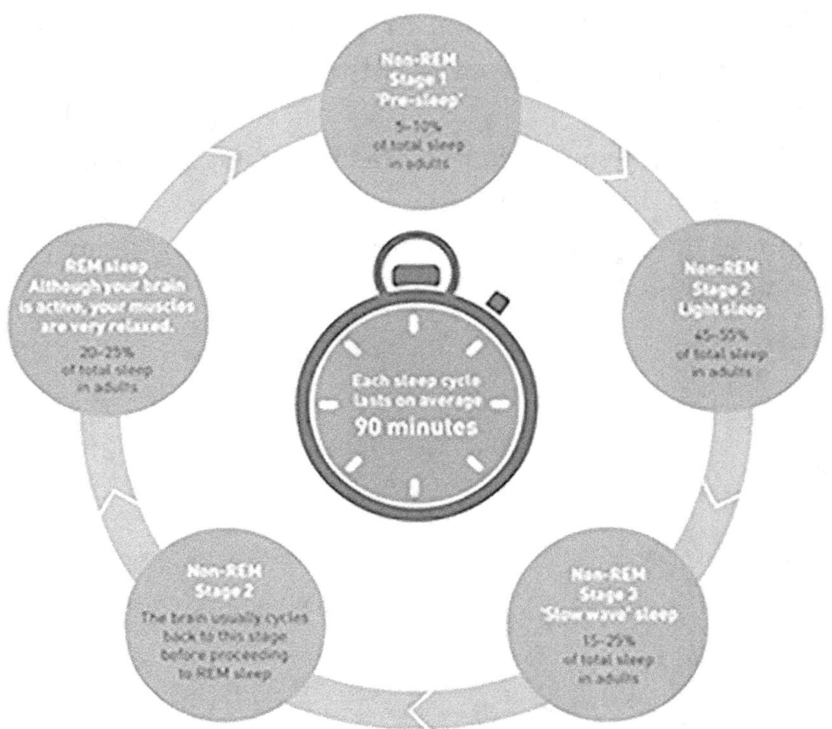

Sleep is a necessity. It allows your brain and body to recover after periods of wakefulness. Specifically, sleep restores your body's ability to function, to repair body tissues, create hormones, consolidate memories and learning, and regulate mood. Sleep makes up such an important part of our lives, that there are people who spend most of their careers dedicated to the topic.

Whether you experience an occasional day of sleepiness, or you feel like you spend most of your days in a sleep-deprived state, it is important to understand the different stages of sleep. This can then help you improve the quality of your sleep so that you will enhance your functioning when you are awake.

No one stage of sleep is more important than another. Studies have shown that each stage plays a distinctive role in your health. In addition, your sleep follows a predictable pattern every night. In other words, actual stages exist where your brain waves change, the ability to be awakened easily changes, and there are specific times when you experience vivid dreaming.

Sleep can be divided into two major categories – **REM sleep and non-REM sleep.**

REM stands for "Rapid Eye Movement."

First, we will discuss **non-REM sleep**, as this is always the starting point for healthy adults when you fall asleep. According to the National Sleep Foundation, three phases of non-REM sleep exist, each lasting from 5 to 15 minutes, and making up about 75% of your sleep at night. You must pass through all three phases before you reach the REM phase about 90 minutes after you first fall asleep. This cycle of non-REM – REM sleep repeats itself throughout the night, with the first full cycle lasting between 70 and 100 minutes. The second and later sleep cycles last between 90 and 120 minutes.

The three phases of non-REM sleep include:

N1 (also known as Stage 1):

Your eyes are closed, and you feel drowsy. Your brain activity starts to slow down. This is the transition period from wakefulness to sleep. During this time, you may experience the sensation of falling, as well as a muscle jerk that wakes you up. This is normal. Muscle tone continues to be high.

In this stage, you are still easily awakened, and you will not feel too drowsy or disoriented if woken up. If awakened from this stage, you may not even be aware that you had fallen asleep. This stage usually lasts no more than seven minutes.

N2 (also known as Stage 2):

Your brain waves become even slower, but they have occasional bursts of activity. Your body temperature goes down. If you are awakened from this stage, you will know that you have been sleeping.

N3 (also known as Stages 3 and 4):

Recordings of your brain waves at these stages demonstrate slow waves called, "delta waves." Your body temperature decreases even more, your breathing is slower, and your blood pressure decreases. This is what is typically known as the "deep sleep" stage.

It is harder to wake someone up during this stage of sleep, but if you are awakened, you will feel groggy, you may feel disoriented, and it will take some time to feel alert.

This restorative stage of sleep is important for your body to recover from the fatigue it undergoes from the previous hours you were awake, and to build up energy for the next day. Your body also rebuilds bone and muscle, repairs tissues, and increases the functioning of your immune system, during this time of sleep. Growth hormone is also released, which is important for muscle development and growth.

Most of Stages 3 and 4 slow-wave sleep occurs in the early hours of the night. In other words, as the night progresses, you spend less and less of your sleep in N3.

REM sleep –

As previously mentioned, REM stands for "rapid eye movement." Your heart rate and breathing increase during REM sleep. Your breathing sounds shallow and irregular. Your eyes move rapidly, hence the term, rapid eye movement. Your muscle tone decreases so significantly that it resembles paralysis.

This stage of sleep typically occurs ninety minutes after you first fall asleep, and approximately every ninety minutes thereafter in your sleep that night. The first REM sleep period lasts no more than ten minutes, and continues to increase each cycle of the night, resulting in being around an hour long for the final REM episode of the night. As a result, most of your REM sleep occurs in the early morning hours. Although dreaming occurs at all stages of sleep, you have the most vivid dreams during REM sleep when the brain is quite active.

You move through all these stages in a sequential manner, repeating the stages as you sleep.

How Much Sleep Do You Need?

The amount of sleep a person needs is dependent upon their age. For example, adults need between seven and nine hours of sleep every night, while children and teenagers need between eight and eleven.

It should come as no shock that newborns need between 14 and 17 hours of sleep every day, while infants can make do with between 12 and 15, toddlers around 11 and 14, and preschoolers 10 and 13. When it comes to school aged children just nine (up to 11) hours are sufficient, and teenagers only need between eight and 10.

Adults of all ages need just seven hours of sleep, though nine is the optimum for younger adults, and eight is for older adults.

If it is not possible for a person to get the full amount, they can at least try at sleeping the minimum number of hours, which in most cases is eight hours. The only time a person should get more than eleven hours of sleep is when they are an infant to one-years-old.

Should a person fail to get the recommended amount of sleep, they should expect to start to feel the consequences. When people don't get the sleep, they need daily, they often say that they will catch up on sleep and decide to sleep for more than the recommended amount of time when they do finally head to bed. There is no such thing as catching up on sleep, so people may want to start making time to get the sleep they need.

The abovementioned consequences of poor sleep are only a few of the many negatives. This should put it in perspective for those who don't believe that a lack of sleep with change the way they function.

With there being so many negative effects of not getting enough sleep, people should strongly consider getting the appropriate amount of sleep. You only have one life to live and if getting a little bit more sleep can help keep you healthy, then why not make this simple change?

Considering that we spend one third of our lives asleep, knowing how much sleep is required is a good question. However, it often comes with an over-generalization.

For example, in March 2015, the National Sleep Foundation came up with some guidelines on how much sleep that people, of different ages, should be getting.

The recommendations were for healthy people with normal sleep patterns. The appropriate duration of sleep for a newborn, for example, is 14 – 17 hours. Whereas, teenagers are reported to be fine with 8 – 10 hours. Young adults and middle-age adults should be aiming for 7 – 9 hours per night, and older adults should try to get 7 – 8 hours of sleep. So, although the duration of sleep varies by age, there is a similarity amongst age groups.

The truth is that sleep is complex and multifactorial. The "magic" number of sleep that you have probably heard the most is "eight hours." Although the National Sleep Foundation came out with these guidelines, some people who work in the field still advocate a more common-sense approach to determining how much sleep you need. This will be discussed in what follows.

If you asked a stranger how much sleep you require, he would probably tell you "eight hours." However, the fact is that this stranger knows nothing about you – about your lifestyle, your job, your stresses. It would be like you trying to determine how many calories the stranger across the street should be consuming every day without you knowing if she exercises, if she is muscle building, or if she is pregnant.

With that in mind, it makes more sense to monitor how you feel, and determine what sleep duration is best for you. You can monitor things like:

How long it takes you to fall asleep – If you fall asleep as soon as your head hits the pillow, then you may need more sleep. If it takes you a long time to fall asleep, then perhaps you are sleeping too much.

Does your body wake up before your alarm? – Your body knows when it is time to wake up. Your internal clock is much wiser than any alarm clock, that you buy, will ever be.

How do you feel during the day? – If you are struggling to keep your eyes open, then you may need more sleep. If you can stay awake and alert, then the amount of sleep you got is probably fine.

By monitoring these things, it can help you adjust your schedule accordingly, so that you get the desired amount of sleep you need.

What Is Insomnia

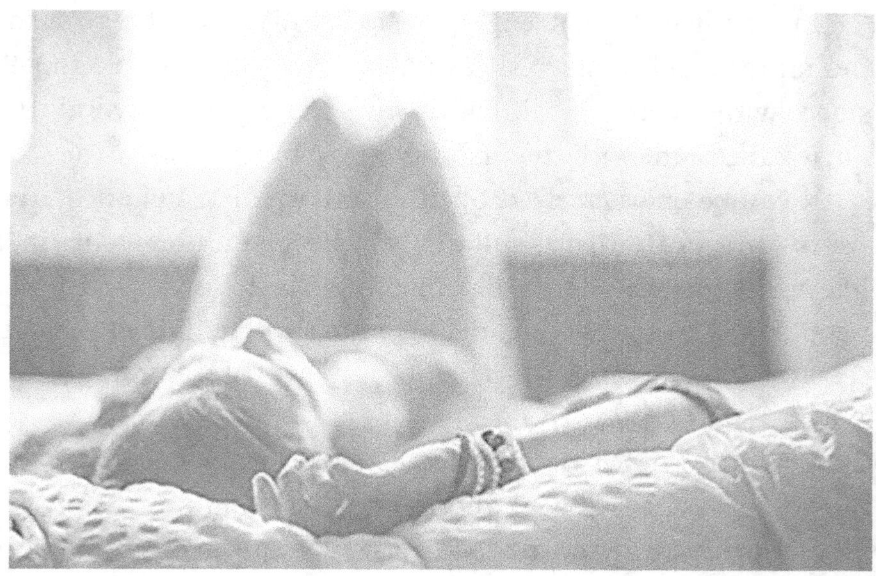

We've all had trouble sleeping from time to time, but what is the difference between that and insomnia?

Insomnia is defined as taking more than 30 minutes to fall asleep, waking up too early, or sleeping less than 6.5 hours a night. Insomnia is two times more common in women than in men and affects 6% to 10% of adults.

Insomnia may be preventing you from falling asleep, or preventing you from staying asleep, even when you have every chance to. Insomniacs feel dissatisfied with the sleep that they are getting, and suffer from a host of symptoms, which may include low energy, decreased performance, fatigue, mood swings, and difficulty concentrating.

Insomnia is the most common sleep disorder and is often undiagnosed and untreated.

Insomnia can involve lying in bed at night, unable to turn off the mind to get to sleep. It can also involve being able to get to sleep without much difficulty but waking up several times during the night with the inability to get back to sleep.

It can be characterized by duration, too. For instance, **acute insomnia is fleeting,** and tends to be a result of events in life, like stressful news, or a big meeting the following day. Many people will experience acute insomnia in their lives, and this resolves itself without the need for any type of treatment.

Types of Insomnia

Primary insomnia indicates sleep problems that are not otherwise associated with another medical condition.

Secondary insomnia occurs because of some other medical condition, including, but not limited to heartburn, depression, chronic pain, medication, or substance abuse.

Insomnia can vary in duration and how often it occurs and is therefore classified as acute or chronic.

Acute Insomnia

Acute insomnia is short term or occasional. Acute forms typically last from one night to a few weeks. Acute insomnia can also come and go, with periods of time when a person has no sleep problems.

Chronic Insomnia

Chronic insomnia lasts a long time and is ongoing. This is characterized by three sleepless nights a week over a period of three months. Typically, insomnia is considered chronic when the sufferer experiences it at least three nights a week for a month or longer.

There are many causes of chronic insomnia. This can include shift work, medications, a change in environment, clinical disorders, and unhealthy sleep habits. Treatment is beneficial to those with chronic insomnia as it can return the sufferer to a healthy pattern of sleep. It is often linked with other issues, though, such as psychiatric issues. In these cases, it can be difficult to determine the underlying cause.

Insomniacs tend to have trouble not only falling asleep, *but also* staying asleep. They may also often wake up too early.

The method of treatment includes medical, behavioral, and psychological components. It is dependent on the patient.

It's a common problem for adults, with around 30% of the population complaining of sleep disrupting. Though, only 10% have the symptoms that are associated with the impairment related to insomnia.

Causes of Chronic Insomnia

The causes of chronic insomnia can be complex and can result from a combination of factors, including, but not limited to:

- Depression (the most common cause of insomnia)
- Chronic pain, such as that from arthritis, fibromyalgia or another illness
- Parkinson's disease
- Chronic stress
- Kidney disease
- Restless leg syndrome

- Pregnancy
- Menopause
- Sleep apnea
- Asthma

Behavioral reasons include:

- Excessive use of alcohol or caffeine before bedtime
- Excessive naps late in the day

Risk Factors and Things That Contribute to Insomnia

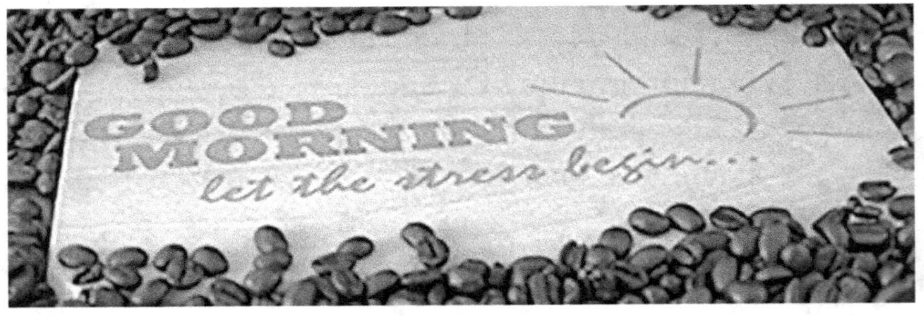

There is a variety of issues that may be contributing to your insomnia, let's look at some of the risk factors.

- **Anxiety**, depression, post traumatic stress disorder, and other mental health conditions increase risk for insomnia.
- **Anxiety & Stress**. Stress is a major contributor to sleepless nights. Mildly stressful events can cause temporary insomnia, while other highly traumatic ones,

such as divorce, death of a loved one or grave financial woes can lead to chronic insomnia.

Worry keeps your mind active. If you are experiencing issues at work, or in your family life, then you may feel anxious. This often results in difficulty sleeping. Additionally, traumatic events such as job loss, divorce, or the loss of someone close to you, can cause chronic anxiety and stress and result in chronic insomnia.

- **Depression**. These two go hand in hand, with depression being one of insomnia's most common sources. This could be related to a chemical imbalance, or that you're having troubling thoughts, which are stopping you from falling asleep. Other common mental health issues related to insomnia include anxiety, bipolar disorder, and PTSD.

- **Sex**. Women suffer from insomnia at twice the rate of men. Woman experience a variety of hormone shifts throughout their life, from menstrual cycles to pregnancy and menopause. Insomnia is common for women who are about to go through menopause. This period, known as perimenopause, is also accompanied by hot flashes and night sweats. According to experts, women in the postmenopausal stage of life struggle to sleep due to a lack of estrogen in the system.

- **Age**. Due to changes in sleep patterns and health, insomnia increases in those ages 60 or older. Older adults tend to struggle to enjoy a sustained sleep during an eight-hour sleep cycle. To make up for this, they may need to find time to nap in the afternoon. The Mayo Clinic estimates that almost 50% of people over 60 deals with insomnia symptoms.

- **Medication**. There is a variety of medications, both prescription and over the counter that can result in insomnia. Products like decongestants, weight loss supplements, and pain medications often contain caffeine. While an antihistamine may leave you feeling drowsy, unfortunately they also result in frequent urination, which will only serve to disturb your sleep. The prescription medications that often cause sleep disruptions include stimulants, antidepressants, allergy medications, and heart and blood pressure medicines.

- **Stimulants**. Energy drinks, coffee, tea, and soft drinks all contain caffeine, thus are considered stimulants. This can interfere with your ability to sleep. If you are guilty of enjoying these stimulants *and* you have difficulty sleeping, you should avoid these products after 2pm. Switch to decaf. Another stimulant is nicotine. Meanwhile, alcohol may be a sedative, but it prevents deep stages of sleep. Therefore, you might nod off quickly, but you will toss and turn, making your rest inadequate.

- **Medical conditions**. There is a variety of medical conditions that can trigger insomnia. The chronic medical conditions that are often tied to sleep issues include arthritis, breathing issues, diabetes, chronic pain, sleep apnea, frequent urination, cardiovascular disease, cancer, menopause, gastroesophageal reflux disease, obesity, overactive thyroid, and frequent urination.

- **Obesity**. The CDC suggests that obesity is linked to many sleep disorders. Adults who get less than six hours of sleep a night tend to have a 33% obesity rate. Yet, that number is just 22% for those getting at least seven hours of sleep a night. This pattern holds true for both women and men, across every age group and ethnicity.

- **Sleep disorders**. There are a few common sleep disorders when can disturb sleep. A great example would be sleep apnea. This is characterized by pauses in breathing, as well as loud snoring. Another example would be restless leg syndrome. The reason this disturbs sleep is because it is accompanied by a crawling sensation in the legs. This can only be relived through movement, thus the disturbance.

- **Environmental Changes**. Your body's circadian rhythm can be disturbed by long distance travel, as well as by shift work. Your circadian rhythm is a cycle that is controlled by sunlight. It's your internal clock and it regulates your metabolism, body temperature, and of course, your sleep cycles.

- **Sleep habits**. When you are worried about not being able to sleep, it becomes infinitely more difficult to get to sleep. If you're having sleep issues, try out the following tips to ease your way into sleep: a bubble bath before bed, don't work in bed, don't watch TV in bed, enjoy soothing music, avoid eating before bed. Avoid looking at any screens at least 30 minutes before bed.
- **Working night shifts** or changing work shifts frequently can lead to insomnia.
- **Jet lag** from regular travel across multiple time zones can cause insomnia.

Diagnosing Insomnia

An evaluation that includes a physical exam, medical history, and a sleep history is used to diagnose insomnia. Sometimes patients are asked to keep a sleep diary to track sleep patterns. For serious and chronic insomnia, a referral to a sleep center for special tests may be given.

Complications of Insomnia

- Insomnia has been linked to high blood pressure, congestive heart failure, diabetes, and other ailments.
- Insomnia can affect performance on the job or at school.
- Slowed reaction time increases risk of accidents while driving, or at work.

- Psychiatric problems, such as depression and anxiety can result from chronic or acute insomnia.
- Overweight or obesity is a common result of insomnia.
- Irritability and fatigue is often seen after sleepless nights.
- Complications in work and social relationships are also common.
- Substance abuse can result when one suffers from insomnia on a regular basis.
- One of the biggest issues with abnormal sleep patterns is that the individual who doesn't get adequate rest becomes sleep deprived, which results in the inability to perform the normal activities of daily living. Sleep deprivation can also affect memory, focus, and cognition.

Why is Sleep So Important for Your Health?

You already know that sleep is important. Without adequate amounts, you feel sleepy. You may also experience other obvious signs and symptoms such as crankiness, headaches, and/or trouble concentrating. However, there are even more serious consequences of not getting enough shut-eye. These are explained in what follows:

Your Physical Health –

1. Increased Risk of Obesity due to the following factors –

a.) No energy – If you do not get adequate sleep at night, you may delay getting out of bed in the morning, because you are too sleepy. As a result, now you do not have enough time to make a healthy breakfast and pack a healthy lunch. You rush out of the house, and you pick up a coffee and donut on the way to work. If you packed a lunch, you eat whatever you threw together at the last minute in the morning, or you buy whatever is on the menu at the cafeteria that day. On your way home, you are tired, and you do not feel like spending an hour in the kitchen preparing something, so you decide to get take-out pizza. You decide to skip the gym that night, because you are just too tired.

You can see how this becomes a vicious cycle and can result in weight gain.

b.) Your body's use of glucose is impaired – Normally, when you eat, your body's cells are supposed to use the energy (glucose). However, when you are sleep deprived, your body is not as efficient at doing this. This makes you feel more tired, hungrier so you eat more, and it also increases your chance of diabetes.

c.) Your hormones are thrown out-of-whack – A hormone called, cortisol, is produced by your adrenal glands. It is commonly referred to as one of the "stress hormones." Cortisol increases with lack of sleep, and it also makes it harder to sleep. Normally, your cortisol levels should be highest in the morning so that it is easy to wake up, and lowest in the evenings when your body prepares for sleep and as it sleeps. High levels of cortisol, when it should be low in your body, is linked to weight gain, obesity, and diabetes.

A couple other important hormones that are affected by lack of sleep include grehlin and leptin. Grehlin is the hormone that tells you when you are hungry, and that it is time to eat. In contrast, leptin is a hormone that tells you when you are full, and that it is time to stop eating. Unfortunately, when you don't get enough sleep, grehlin increases and leptin decreases, putting you at risk of weight gain.

2. **Increased Risk of Diseases** – As already mentioned above, lack of sleep increases potential for weight gain and unstable blood sugars, which then increases your risk of diabetes.

Heart disease is also higher if you are chronically sleep deprived. According to the National Sleep Foundation, despite exercise, age, weight, and smoking habits, your risk of heart disease goes up if you do not get enough sleep. Although the exact causes are not known, lack of sleep is linked to high blood pressure, high cholesterol, and increased inflammation in the body. All sleep-deprived individuals are at risk of this, but people with sleep apnea tend to have even higher rates of heart disease than those without the medical problem.

3. **Lowered Immune System Functioning** – Your immune system is what protects your body from germs. When your body encounters germs, your body goes to work to fight off the invaders. However, when you don't get enough sleep, your immune system does not function as well, increasing your susceptibility to colds, flu, and other ailments. The simple explanation is that your immune system cannot produce the germ-fighting cells that it needs when you aren't getting enough sleep. Your body is effective at restoring these fighter cells when you sleep.

4. **Your Sex Life Suffers** – This could have been included in the topic of hormone disruption above. This is because the sex hormone, testosterone, is reduced in men and women who are leading sleep-deprived lives. This, in turn, results in a decreased interest in sex for both genders, erectile dysfunction in males, and reduced vaginal lubrication in females.

5. **Increased Risk of Injuries and Accidents** – When you are tired, your concentration and focus is poor. Therefore, this puts you at increased risk of workplace injuries and car accidents.

Your Cognitive, Mental, & Emotional Health –

Pulling all-nighters is not only a bad idea for your physical health, it also negatively impacts your mental, cognitive, and emotional health. More people are recognizing that the days of bragging about being able to function with only a few hours of sleep, is really a health hazard and not something with which to mess around.

Here are 7 ways that sleep deprivation affects these areas of your health:

1. **Altered Mood** – You already know that you feel irritable and short-tempered when you don't get enough sleep. Chronic lack of sleep, however, also increases your chances of depression and anxiety.

2. **Decreased Ability to Handle Stress** – Stressful situations are difficult enough to handle when you have gotten a good sleep. When you get less than ideal amounts of sleep, and you are dealing with stress, your ability to do this well, deteriorates significantly. You may get angry, yell, cry, or do things that you normally wouldn't do if you had gotten a good night of sleep.

3. **Decreased Ability to Think & Learn** – Your ability to concentrate and focus on tasks, make decisions, and carry through with them, is hampered a great deal with lack of sleep.

In addition, your ability to learn new things is also reduced. Sleep is known to help with new learning, and it is probably the reason why babies and young children sleep so much as they are constantly learning and adapting to their environments. New learning does not end with childhood, so adequate sleep continues to play an important role in adults. In addition, your brain assimilates information as you sleep, helping you to retain information.

4. **Reduced Judgment Skills** – Although this also falls under the inability to think, it deserves its own bullet point. If your judgment and insight is lacking due to poor sleep, your decision-making skills will be affected. You may make more impulsive decisions, or do things that are potentially unsafe while driving, for example. Your ability to assess situations accurately decreases.

5. **Negatively Impacts Relationships** – Because of your reduced ability to handle stress and your increased irritability, it makes sense that your personal and work relationships will suffer. This may also take a toll on your self-esteem as friendships and relationships are ruined, and you find that you have no one with which to talk.

6. **Poor Memory** – Again, this goes back to the inability to concentrate and focus on what is happening around you. If you do not register things in your short-term memory, it is impossible for the brain to convert memories to long term ones.

7. **Slowed Reaction Time** – Sleepiness when driving, has been described as dangerous as driving under the

influence of alcohol. If you mix lack of sleep and alcohol, it makes you even more dangerous behind the wheel.

Not only is driving dangerous when you lack sleep, working in certain industries or professions, when sleep-deprived, can be extremely dangerous. For example, construction workers and police officers are two of many professions that require alertness and the ability to react quickly.

5 Ways to Make Sleep a Priority

Hopefully, the importance of sleep and how it impacts your physical and mental well-being is becoming clear. With that being said, you need to make sleep a priority. Think about how much better you will feel, and what you can accomplish if you work on improving your sleep.

6 Ways to Make Your Sleep a Priority

1. Establish a bedtime routine: **Start getting ready at least one hour before you plan to go to bed. Have a light snack, a bath, & put on your pajamas.**

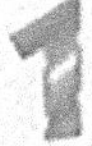

2. Set up a pleasant atmosphere: **Set your bedroom up so that it is cozy & you enjoy retreating to it at the end of the day.**

3. Recognize if you are productive or just keeping busy: **If you are checking your email for the 15th time that day, perhaps you need to re-evaluate what the purpose is for doing certain things.**

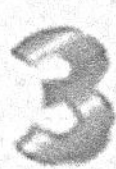

4. Remind yourself that "Rome wasn't built in a day": **Realize that there will always be things that don't get done in a day, and that you can start fresh the next day after a good night of sleep.**

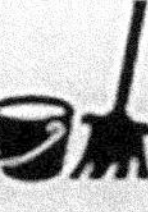

5. Avoid emotional & financial conversations before bedtime: **Reserve difficult & stressful conversations for daytime when you're most alert.**

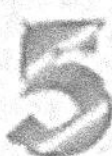

6. Remember that sleep IS important: **Sleep is as important as healthy eating and exercise. You can not skimp on sleep AND yet have good health.**

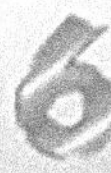

You CAN Improve Your Sleep!

If your sleep does not improve, no matter what you try, you should speak to your doctor as there could be underlying medical or psychological problems.

Here are some tips on how to learn to prioritize your sleep, and how to get to bed at a reasonable hour:

1. **Establish a bedtime routine** – Just as children benefit from routines, so do adults. It is beneficial to create a routine where you start getting ready at least an hour before lights out. This may include having a bath (not too hot though as this will impede falling asleep), getting into your pajamas, having a light snack, and reading a book.

2. **Set up a pleasant atmosphere** – You want to set up your bedroom so that it is cozy, and so that you enjoy retreating to it at the end of a busy day. Pay attention to the colors of your walls. Choose calming, soothing paint colors such as soft grays, lavender, or sage. Set up a lamp with a soft yellow or red light. Avoid lights that emit blue wavelengths. Decorate your walls in such a way that it adds to the beauty of the room.

3. **Recognize the difference between being busy and being productive** – Have you ever found yourself wasting time at the end of the day, because you are tired, but it feels like it is too early to go to bed? For example,

you might be surfing the internet or checking your emails for the 15th time that day, but you aren't doing anything productive. Instead, you are just keeping yourself busy. Learn to recognize when you are doing this, so that you can spend your time more wisely, and you don't steal time from your bedtime routine.

4. **Remind yourself of this saying, "Rome wasn't built in a day."** - When you look around your house at the end of the day, you can always find something else to do before you head off to bed – dirty dishes in the sink, crumbs on the floor that need to be swept, or another email waiting to be answered. This is never going to change. Realize that there will always be things that don't get done in a day, and that you can start fresh the next day after a good night of sleep.

5. **Avoid emotional and financial conversations before bedtime** – Evenings are not a good time to be having difficult conversations with friends or family. Talking about your financial situation, such as your outstanding credit card balance, should also not be done before bedtime. Instead, these conversations, including texts and emails, should be reserved for daytime when you have the energy, and when they are not going to cause you extra stress right before it is time to fall asleep.

6 Tips to Improve Your Sleep Tonight

Sleep hygiene involves doing several different things that prepare your body for sleep and allow it to have quality sleep so that you can be alert the next day. Following a regular bedtime routine is one aspect of sleep hygiene, but there are many other things that you can do to improve your sleep starting now. These include:

1. **Caffeine cut-off times** – You know that caffeine should be limited before bedtime, but when exactly in the day should you stop drinking caffeinated beverages? It is probably earlier than you realize. A general guideline is no later than 2 p.m. This is because studies have shown that consumption of caffeine even six hours before bedtime, can cause disturbances in sleep quality. Although you may not notice the effects of the caffeine when you go to sleep, your body's sleep quality will still be poorer.

   Therefore, recommendations include drinking caffeinated beverages in the morning hours, and very early afternoon. Drink no more than 400 mg of caffeine per day, which is equal to about 4 cups of coffee. Any more than that, and you should be choosing decaffeinated coffee or tea. And don't forget that caffeine is also found in cola, hot chocolate, cocoa, and some over-the-counter and prescription pain medications.

2. **Limit alcohol intake** – Although alcohol is a central nervous system depressant, and causes you to feel sleepy, it disrupts your sleep quality. Your body does not enter the deeper sleep cycle, which is necessary to restore your energy for the next day. In addition, as the alcohol wears off, your brain "reboots" causing disruption in the normal brain wave pattern that allows for quality sleep.

3. **Go to bed at the same time every night – give or take 20 minutes.** You have, no doubt, heard this advice before. By doing so, you can train your body to wake up without an alarm.

4. **Have sex before sleep time** – Sleep hygiene experts tell you to reserve your bed only for sleep and sex. However, let's take it a step further. Studies show that sex, in conjunction with orgasms, is a great way to end the day before you nod off. This is because sex can distract you (be sure to put away your phone and other electronic devices!), and it promotes the release of "feel-good" hormones that relax you and reduce your perception of pain.

5. **Set up your bedroom environment** – In addition to setting up a pleasant setting that is cozy and has calming colors, you need to limit the light in your bedroom before you fall asleep and during sleep. Even the light from your alarm clock can negatively affect your sleep, so cover the light emitting from it. In addition, be sure to use room-

darkening shades over the windows. Keep the room quiet. If you live on a busy, loud street, for example, you may need to create white noise using a fan, or you can use an app. Just be sure that, if it is a fan, that it is not blowing directly on you. Keep your bedroom temperature lower, as this will promote better sleep.

6. **Get up after 20 minutes in bed, if you haven't fallen asleep yet** – There is no point to staying in bed tossing and turning. All it does it frustrate you, which impedes the goal – falling asleep. Instead, it is better to get up and do something quiet. The goal remains the same. You want to get back to bed and get some sleep. Try taking your mind off the issue by reading a book (not a tablet or smartphone as the blue light emitted will increase your wakefulness), meditating, listening to calming music, or doing some relaxation exercises.

What Does Your Biological Clock Have to do With Your Sleep?

We all have a biological clock. This biological clock is sometimes referred to as your circadian rhythm, or your sleep-wake cycle. In fact, there is a small "part" in your brain that controls all of this. It controls when your brain and other organs secrete chemical messengers, known as hormones to other parts of your body to cause things to happen in your body. Even when this part is removed from the brain, it continues to function all on its own!

The reason that it is important to have a general understanding of how this biological clock works, is so that you can understand HOW to improve your sleep. If you understand some of the hormones involved, for example, it will help you know whether you should be using natural supplements to help your sleep. In what follows, you will learn more about two specific hormones (melatonin and cortisol) and a compound (adenosine) that are important for your sleep, and how they play an important role in the functioning of your biological clock.

Melatonin -

Melatonin is a hormone that is produced in your brain. It is synthesized from another hormone in your brain called serotonin. Melatonin production is stimulated by darkness, or when blue light is no longer entering your eyes. It is one hormone that contributes to feeling sleepy. It is also known to play a role in the reduction of aging in your brain and body, as well as to have cancer-fighting properties.

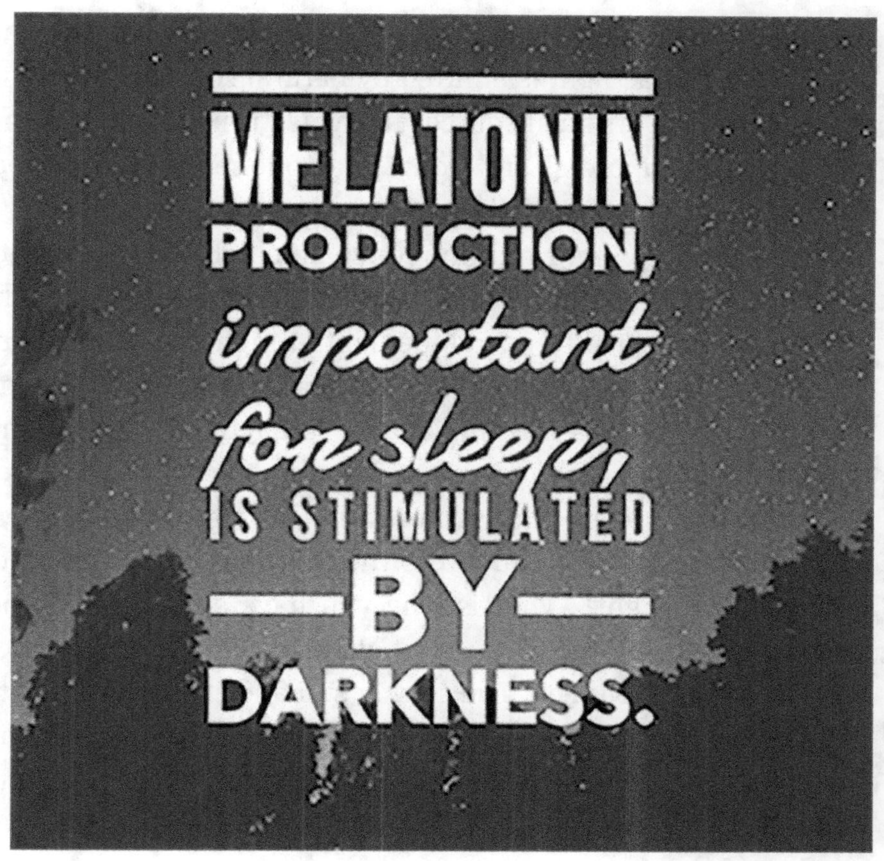

Melatonin production comes to a halt when blue light enters your eyes by way of daylight. When your brain sense blue light, melatonin production stops. As an aside, these blue wavelengths are what make the sky look blue when it scatters in the atmosphere. It is also important to note that special "daylight lamps", used by people with Seasonal Affective Disorder (SAD) or the "winter blues", also provide the eyes with blue light required to elevate mood and reduce the fatigue associated with this disorder.

As you can see, blue light is what regulates your wake and sleep cycles. Blue light is emitted by natural sources such as the sun, but also by artificial sources from electronic devices such as televisions, computers, and your smartphone, as well as most household and workplace lights.

It is therefore important to reduce blue light exposure in the evenings and while you sleep, to get quality sleep. Our bodies were never designed to need blue light at nighttime, but the use of artificial light sources has made it nearly impossible to avoid. Your body continues to think that it is daytime, and does not produce adequate volumes of melatonin, thus confusing your body's natural cycles. This is a modern-day issue, because years ago, lanterns and oil lamps were the norm and these items did not emit blue light. That is why you have some of your best sleeps when camping, if you pay attention not to use artificial lighting in the evenings. The setting sun and the natural light of the fire do not interfere with your body's biological clock and encourage it to do what it's supposed to do – release melatonin required for sleep.

Cortisol –

This is another important hormone that affects your sleep. Under normal, healthy conditions, cortisol levels should rise in the mornings, and decrease in the evenings. In contrast, the sleep hormone, melatonin, is supposed to rise in the evenings when darkness prevails and decrease in the mornings for waking. So as melatonin levels decrease, your cortisol levels pick up. Both hormones are similar though, in that they both work on an approximate 24-hour cycle in your body, supporting your body's biological clock.

Cortisol is known as one of the "fight or flight stress hormones." It is released by your adrenal glands in your body. When released, cortisol increases your blood sugar levels, so that your muscles and brain get the energy needed to act. It helps wake you up, and keeps you alert during the daytime. It is typically highest at 8 a.m., and lowest between the hours of midnight and 4 a.m. Unfortunately, too much cortisol is not a good thing either, especially when your cortisol levels remain high throughout the evening. This occurs when you are experiencing emotional or physical (i.e. sickness) stress. Even having an upsetting conversation, learning of exciting news, or watching a thrilling television show in the evening, can increase your cortisol levels. These elevated cortisol levels in the evenings can then keep you from falling asleep and prevent you from having a restful sleep.

Unfortunately, if your adrenal glands continue to secrete cortisol, as is the case during periods of prolonged stress, eventually they burn out (this is what is referred to as "adrenal fatigue"), and normal surges of cortisol in the morning no longer occur. In fact, if your adrenal glands are no longer producing adequate volumes of cortisol, your blood sugars levels are not going to be high enough at nighttime, so your sleep will suffer as you wake up earlier from the brain signaling its hunger.

To complicate matters, if you do not get enough sleep one night, your cortisol levels will be elevated the next night.

As you can see, your body's systems and hormones are all inter-related. What happens to one, affects another, and together, they impact the quality and quantity of your sleep.

Adenosine –

This is another chemical naturally found in your body. Without getting into the complex chemistry, all you need to know is that adenosine builds up each hour that you are awake causing you to become sleepy. Adenosine is a byproduct of your cells working and using energy in your body. It works in conjunction with melatonin, which is released in response to darkness. Adenosine breaks down when you sleep.

It is believed that when you exert more energy through physical exercise and physical labor, that your adenosine levels build up more, causing you to feel sleepier at nighttime. That is why you notice feeling very sleepy after a long day of skiing or surfing, for example, compared to when you exert less energy during the day.

7 Ways to Avoid Blue Light at Night

Perhaps you are doing your best to take care of your body - eating healthy foods, getting regular exercise, and reducing your stress levels. Sleep is also part of a healthy lifestyle – both quantity and quality. Studies, however, show that people are sleeping less. One of the reasons for this is the exposure to blue light at the wrong time of day.

Blue light is found in the sun (as well as other color wavelengths). Blue light has a shorter wavelength, and it is energizing and mood enhancing. When this light hits your eyes in the mornings, it sends signals to your brain telling you that it is time to wake up. This is controlled by melatonin production being turned off. Whereas, when the sun sets, you are not exposed to its blue light until sunrise again.

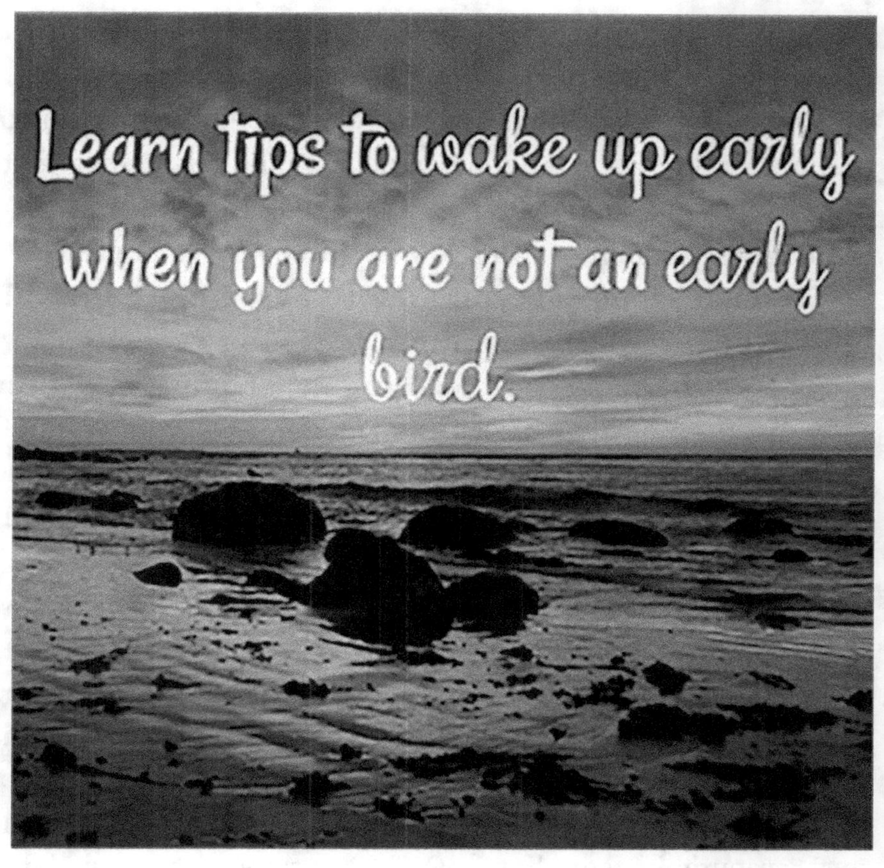

Unfortunately, you continue to be exposed to blue light even when the sun sets. This is because of artificial lighting and technology (TV's, computers, tablets, etc.) in your home. The invention of the light bulb and other technology has tricked your brain into thinking that it is still daytime. It results in increasing your evening alertness, as well as changing your body's biological clock (also referred to as the circadian rhythm) and hormones so that sleep is delayed. In fact, any artificial light exposure in the evening is an issue. Even dim lamps can emit enough blue light to disrupt your sleep rhythms!

Obviously, it is difficult to survive in today's world in total evening darkness. You could read by candlelight, but that is probably not possible when you have worked all day and have evening responsibilities with your children, for example.

So what steps can you take to avoid or reduce blue light exposure in the evening?

1. **Avoid the use of technology at least two hours before bedtime.** This means not using your computer, tablet, smartphone, and television, for example. These items all emit blue light, and prevent the production of melatonin, the latter which is needed to cause you to become sleepy.

2. **If you absolutely must use technology or to be in bright light in the evening, use blue-blocking glasses.** These can also be useful for evening and nightshift workers. Be sure you buy them from a reputable supplier. Your optometrist may be an invaluable resource to make specific recommendations. You can also find them sold online through various outlets.

3. **Maximize exposure to light during the day.** This does not mean sit in the sun all day, otherwise you will potentially end up with other serious problems such as skin cancer or damage to your eyes (cataracts and age-related macular degeneration are accelerated by too

much blue light exposure). Instead, it appears that maximum daytime exposure results in lessening the effects of being exposed to light at night. Plan to take a walk outdoors over your lunch break at the same time every day. This same-day exposure to sunlight can aid your body's internal clock.

In winter, or if you spend days at work with no exposure to natural light, be sure to use a lightbox that provides you with plenty of blue light. You can use it before you go to work, while you are eating your breakfast or applying your cosmetics, for example. If you sit at a desk, you can use a lightbox at work.

4. **You can adjust the colors of your screens on your smartphones, computers, and tablets to warmer, shorter wavelengths.** Set it up so that it happens automatically every evening, and results in less to no exposure to blue light at this time.

5. **Choose lightbulbs that emit less or no blue light** and emit more reddish or warmer hues.

6. **During sleep, cover any lights on your alarm clock or other devices at night.** Use room-darkening shades to avoid exposure from streetlights or your neighbor's lights. Wear a sleep mask.

7. **Go camping** – Whether you like camping or not, this is one of the best ways to avoid blue light exposure at night. It is also a great way to reset your body's biological clock. Therefore, you may want to rethink your family vacation this year. If you are looking for a restful vacation, camping may be the best way to go about getting that.

Recommendations for Artificial Lighting for Quality Sleep – Say What?

Artificial lighting is a norm in modern-day society. When the sun sets, the lights also go on in homes and businesses across the world. Even though studies are demonstrating the importance of limiting exposure to light (blue, in particular) before bedtime, it is highly unlikely that people are going to adopt "lightless" evenings or start using oil lamps or candles again.

Even NASA recognized that the fluorescent lighting on the International Space Station, was disrupting the sleep of astronauts. NASA has since changed the bulbs to ones that do not emit blue light all night.

This begs another question. If you are going to be exposed to light in the evenings, what should you know about lightbulbs to make better choices that have a less-negative impact on your sleep?

Red lightbulbs – You know that blue light disrupts your hormones and sleep levels. Red light, on the other hand, is conducive to good sleep. These are the best lights to use in your bedroom, and for reading a paper book. Red nightlights are also available, if you need to use one in a sleeping area. You can buy them online, at Amazon, for example.

Incandescent lightbulbs – These are the type of bulbs that Thomas Edison brought to the marketplace. Until recent years, these were the most popular bulbs used in homes across North America. Some countries no longer use them, mostly because they are less energy efficient. They also do not last as long – around 1000 hours - as other types created in more recent years. However, they do produce warmer hues, and although not as good as red lightbulbs, they are an option for cutting down on blue light. Keep reading for other options though.

Compact Fluorescent Lighting (CFL's) – You will recognize these lights by the bulbs that are spiral-shaped in appearance. They emit a lot of blue light, and they are a cause of concern for environmental groups related to their mercury content, and how to dispose of them safely. They became popular though as they are more energy efficient, and last longer than incandescent bulbs. These are the bulbs that take a while to get bright when switched on.

Light-Emitting Diodes (LED's) – These bulbs have become even more popular as they are even more energy efficient than CFL's, and they get bright immediately. However, regular LED lightbulbs can emit blue light, and disrupt sleep patterns.

Fortunately, as science is proving the need to eliminate blue light before bedtime and during sleep, some companies are listening. General Electric, for example, has created their "GE Align" lighting. These LED's are designed so as not to disrupt the body's natural sleep rhythms. They do this by controlling how much blue light is emitted. They have AM bulbs meant to be like daylight, which helps to suppress melatonin production. On the other hand, the PM bulbs have an amber light that is like the light of candles and campfires. In this way, they do not disrupt your evening melatonin production needed for quality sleep.

Lighting Science is another company that takes pride in the creation of bulbs for both your home and your body. Its "Goodnight" Sleep-Enhancing bulbs use the same technology as was created for the NASA astronauts.

SCS Lighting Solutions, another company, create the "Sleep Ready Light Bulb," and offer the perfect option for your bedside lamp.

All these bulbs are available for sale at places such as Amazon. In addition, most or all companies offer a daytime option, which can help increase your alertness when you wake up by suppressing melatonin production.

Reduce Your Temperature, Get a Better Sleep

Studies are showing that quality sleep is as important to your health as eating well, exercising, not smoking, and so forth. Sleep is a complex, restorative process. Your body controls the release of hormones and substances that help you sleep. However, many aspects of good sleep are also in your control and require your participation. The use of proper artificial lighting in your home is one way that you can control the quality of sleep you get every night. However, there are other things, related to your body's temperature, that can also be done to prepare your body for a good night of sleep. In what follows, are some of those ideas.

Have you ever tried to sleep after a hot shower or bath, or even in a bedroom that is too warm? You undoubtedly know that this makes it more difficult to fall asleep, and it is also harder to remain sleeping.

In preparation for good sleep, your body's internal temperature must drop about a degree. This normally starts to occur around 90 to 120 minutes before sleep is to occur. Fortunately, in most circumstances, you can manipulate your body's temperature. Knowing this, here is what you need to do to allow this to happen:

- **Avoid hot showers and hot baths right before bed** – Keep the temperature of the water from warm to cool. In fact, in summer, take a cooler shower or go for a cool swim. If possible, go to bed with wet hair, as this will keep your body cooler and improve your sleep.

- **Avoid exercising right before bed** – This is something that you have always heard, but do you really know why this is an issue? It is because, not only does exercise stimulate you, it will also make you feel excessively warm to sleep. If possible, try to exercise earlier in the day. If that is not an option, and it often isn't for everyone, then you can help your body cool itself by taking a cool shower after your exercise workout.

- **Avoid excessive clothing before and at bedtime –** Another way to help your body cool down in the evenings, is to leave your arms and legs exposed. Think boxer shorts for guys, and light nightgowns for females. If you like wearing a fuzzy onesie to sleep, then reduce some of the bedding, or you will negatively affect your ability to fall asleep and to stay asleep.

- **Don't use hot water bottles and heating pads close to bedtime –** The same applies to too much bedding. In colder climates, if you want to warm up your bed before getting in, then put a heading pad in it for a few minutes before you get in, but then turn it off. Otherwise, its heat is bound to wake you up later.

- **Lower the temperature in your home –** With timers on thermostats, you can set the temperature in your home to be lowered a couple hours before bedtime. This will also help with reducing your core body temperature, making it easier to fall asleep, and stay asleep.

While you sleep, aim for a room temperature of no higher than 70 degrees F. 65 degrees F seems to be the most ideal, but you may have to experiment to find what suits your sleep the best.

3 *Things to Consider Before Taking Sleeping Pills*

Sleep is a natural process, but it seems so hard to get sometimes, and you may feel desperate. That is why the pharmaceutical companies keep coming up with new medications for sleep. However, sleeping medications (prescription and non-prescription) should not be your first go-to, if you suddenly find yourself having difficulty falling asleep or maintaining your sleep. This is a discussion that will need to occur with your medical doctor, who knows your medical history and lifestyle challenges.

Before deciding that sleeping pills are required, here are some things to ask yourself first:

1. **Are you looking for short-term results?**
   Over-the-counter or prescription sleeping medications may help you in the short-term, but you are not really fixing the root cause of your sleeping problems. For example, sleeping medications may help with temporary issues such as jet lag, or adjusting to a shift change at work, but they should never be a long-term solution.
   Of concern is that some sleeping medications result in dependence. The side effects of the medications can also be problematic. For example, the effects of the medication may not wear off before morning, making it unsafe to drive with the medication still in your body.

Some people have also been known to do things while under the influence of sleeping medications, such as eating, texting, and even having sex while asleep!

2. **Have you tried making lifestyle changes?**
   Many sleeping issues can be resolved or improved significantly simply by adjusting your lifestyle and your environment. For example, you can learn to control when and how much blue light exposure you get, thus affecting your sleep hormones. This applies to getting adequate daylight, and avoiding computer screens, tablets, etc. before bedtime.

   You can also implement ways that bring your core body temperature down, a necessity to falling asleep. By using stress-reduction techniques, such as meditation, yoga, and deep breathing exercises, you can also learn to sleep better. Other techniques include waking up at the same time every day, getting enough physical exercise in the day, and not drinking caffeine at least six hours before you go to sleep.

3. **Have you tried natural supplements or essential oils for sleeping?**

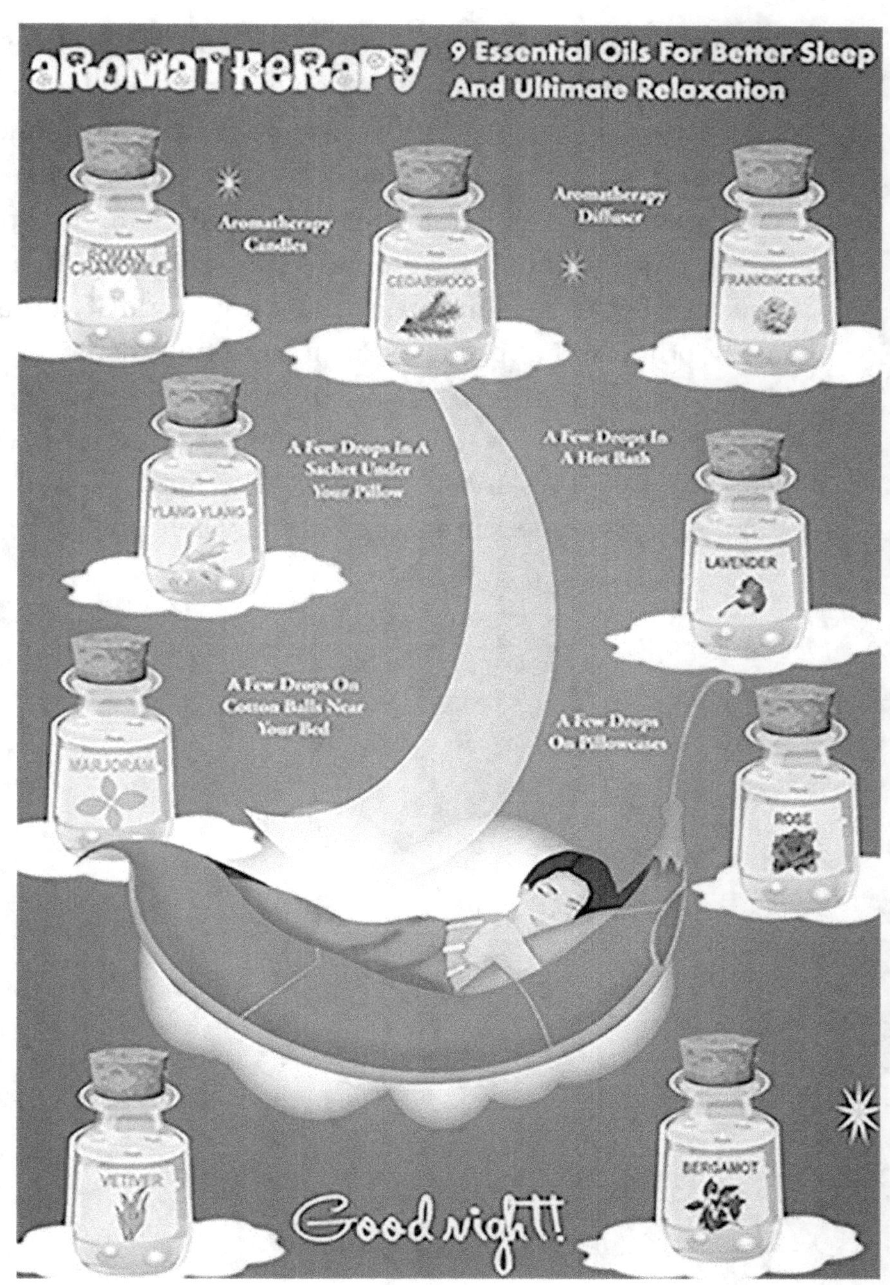
aRoMaTHeRaPy
9 Essential Oils For Better Sleep And Ultimate Relaxation
ROMAN CHAMOMILE
Aromatherapy Candles
CEDARWOOD
Aromatherapy Diffuser
FRANKINCENSE
YLANG YLANG
A Few Drops In A Sachet Under Your Pillow
A Few Drops In A Hot Bath
LAVENDER
A Few Drops On Cotton Balls Near Your Bed
MARJORAM
A Few Drops On Pillowcases
ROSE
VETIVER
Good night!
BERGAMOT

In addition to lifestyle and environmental changes mentioned above, natural supplements and essential oils that promote sleep exist. Because even natural products can exert strong biological effects, it is wise to consult with your physician before starting to use them, or better yet a pharmacist or a naturopathic doctor who can guide you on their use. This is especially important if you are using other herbal products or prescription medications. A naturopathic doctor can be an invaluable resource to educating you on lifestyle habits, changes you can make, as well as the most appropriate suitable natural supplements and essential oils that may help you.

Medical Conditions that Interfere with Normal Sleep

If you are always exhausted, despite making real attempts at improving your sleep, or you have trouble falling asleep or staying asleep (insomnia), then you should always discuss this with your medical doctor. There are two reasons for this. First, some medications contain compounds that make it harder to sleep. For example, some pain medications have caffeine in them. In addition, some asthma medications, and even nasal decongestants can also disrupt your sleep. This is just the tip of the iceberg. Second, several health conditions, both physical or mental, can interfere with your sleep, and some of them can be dangerous.

Here are a few physical medical conditions to know about.

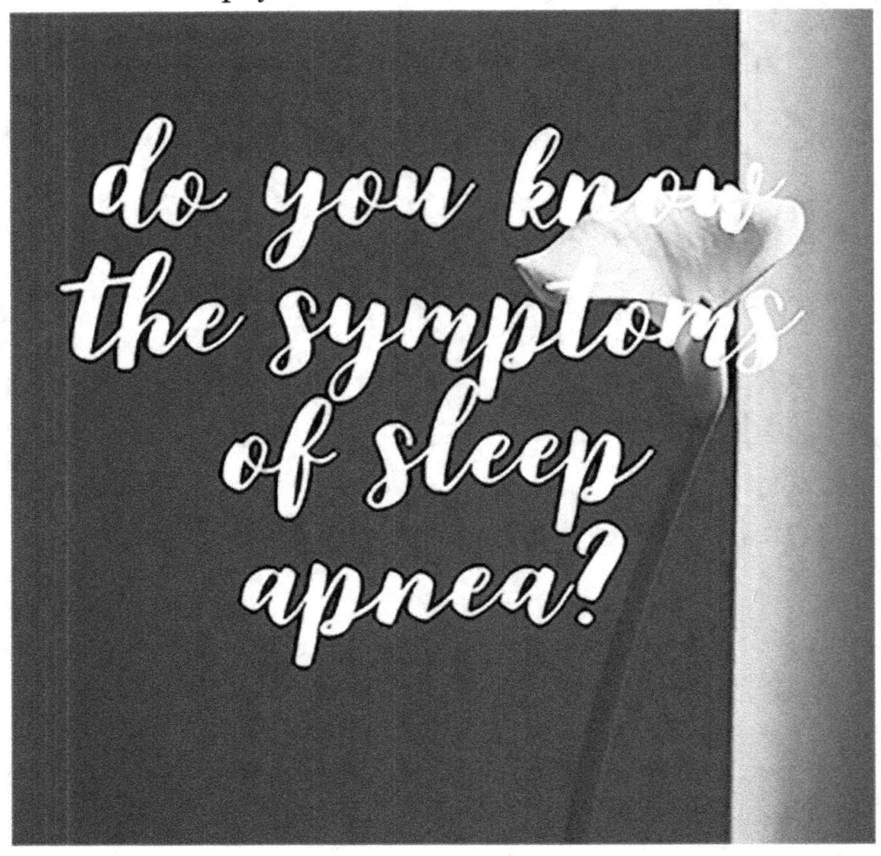

Sleep Apnea – This is actually a very common sleep disorder. Unfortunately, sleep apnea is quite serious, as it involves the interruption of breathing during sleep. Pauses in breathing can last from a few seconds to much longer, and they can occur many times an hour. In one type of sleep apnea, the brain does not send the signals for breathing to occur. The second type of sleep apnea is more common, and it is called "obstructive sleep apnea," because it involves the collapse of tissues in the throat during sleep. It is more common in overweight and obese individuals, and weight loss can be a solution to the problem. However, other things that can contribute to sleep apnea include large tonsils, sinus issues, family history, and so on. So even if you are not overweight, you can still be affected by sleep apnea. In fact, children are also diagnosed with sleep apnea.

Other risk factors for sleep apnea are:
Being of male gender
Being a smoker
You have high blood pressure
You have asthma
You have diabetes
You have reflux/heartburn
You are older than 40
You have nasal blockages from large adenoids, sinus problems, or the bone between your nostrils is offset (deviated nasal septum)

Some of the signs and symptoms that point to the possibility of sleep apnea include:
Choking during sleep
Loud snoring
Morning headaches

Pauses in your breathing while sleeping

Dry mouth when waking up

Exhausted

High blood pressure

Waking up with a dry throat

If you or your partner notice any of the above, be sure to speak to your doctor.

To make a diagnosis, your doctor may order a sleep lab test or a sleep home test to confirm if sleep apnea is the source of your sleep woes. If sleep apnea is confirmed, then your doctor will determine the next step. As previously mentioned, weight loss may be recommended. If large tonsils or adenoids are the issue, then surgery may be the treatment plan. Some people may benefit from special dental appliances or mouth guards that help keep their airway open during sleep. Smoking cessation can also help, as can ensuring you don't sleep on your back. Sewing tennis balls into the back of your pajamas is one way to wake you up if you turn onto your back during sleep. Sometimes, a special machine such as a CPAP (Continuous Positive Airway Pressure) will be recommended to ensure that the tissues in your throat do not collapse during sleep.

Heartburn – Heartburn is the result of regurgitation of stomach contents, including stomach acid, back up your food pipe (the esophagus) that causes a burning pain in your chest. These acidic contents can reach the back of your throat, causing you to cough or choke, and wake up from sleep.

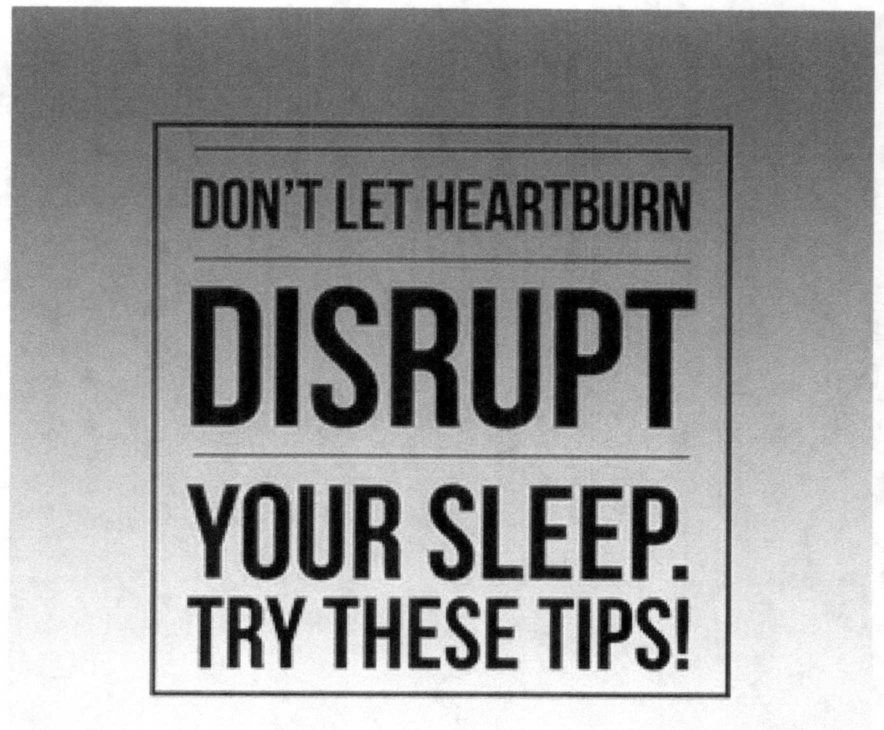

Fortunately, some effective techniques exist to help you manage heartburn, and improve your sleep. These include:

Use a bed wedge – You can find these in medical supply stores that sell all kinds of medical equipment. If they do not have one in stock, they can be ordered in. The purpose for the use of a bed wedge is to raise your upper body on an incline, making it harder for stomach contents to move against gravity. Regular pillows are not effective as you need to raise your chest too.

Sleep on your left side – This is not always effective for people with severe reflux that results in heartburn, but it is worth a try as it works for many. Studies have shown that when you sleep on your left side, there is less chance of stomach contents travelling up your food pipe to your throat when compared to right side lying. Here are two easy sayings to help you remember what side to sleep on: "Right is wrong." or "Left is right."

Elevate the head of your bed – The easiest way to do this is to elevate the head of your bed six inches higher than that of your feet. You can purchase items called "bed blocks" from any medical store, as these are often used by people with arthritis or hip replacements to raise their beds. In the case of heartburn and reflux, you only put the bed blocks under the head of the bed. Like the bed wedge, it makes it harder for stomach acid to make its way upwards against gravity.

Consult with your doctor and a pharmacist – Just as some medications interfere with sleep, some medications also contribute to reflux, causing you to lose quality and quantity of sleep.

Lose a few pounds – By losing weight, you can decrease the severity and frequency of reflux and heartburn.

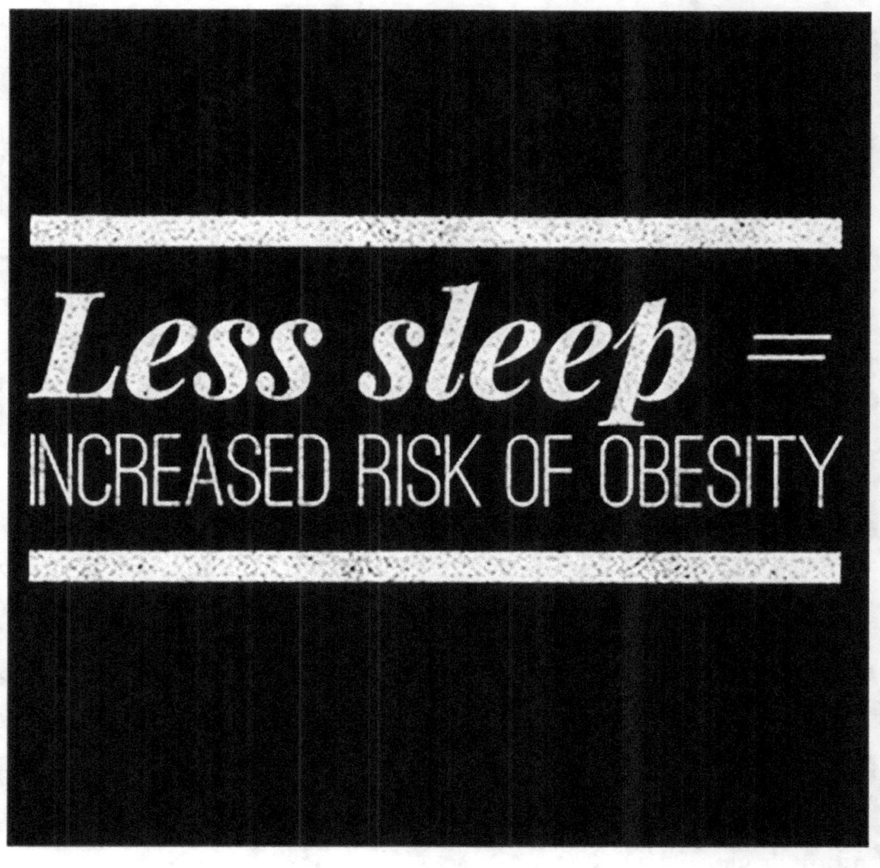

Do not eat a large meal right before bedtime – A small snack is okay to help improve sleep, however you should not be eating a large meal two to three hours before bedtime. In addition, it really is advisable to avoid foods that make your reflux worse. You may need to use a food diary to determine what they are, or you may already know what to avoid. Common culprits are carbonated beverages, coffee, tea, spicy foods, garlic, onions, and fatty fried foods.

Quit smoking – This is much easier said than done. As you know, the average smoker makes many attempts before achieving success. However, it may be worth seeing if giving up the habit also improves your sleep, if it is accompanied by a reduction in reflux symptoms. Smoking is known to relax the muscles of your food pipe (esophagus), contributing to reflux.

Diabètes -

One reason why you may not be sleeping well, is that you have diabetes, and do not even know it. According to the Centers for Disease Control and Prevention, 29 million Americans have diabetes, and ¼ of them don't even know it!

Diabetes and poor sleep go hand in hand. People whose blood sugars are high due to the diabetes, often spend a lot of time up at night having to urinate. They also may wake up with night sweats or wake up due to feelings of low blood sugar (hypoglycemia).

Likewise, poor sleep also increases your risk of diabetes.

If you are diabetic, by eating properly during the day and evening, you can stabilize your blood sugars, so that you will get a better sleep.

Arthritis –

It is estimated that 80% of people with arthritis also suffer from sleep problems. Pain in joints can make it difficult to find a comfortable position to fall asleep and to remain sleeping.

Thyroid Problems –

Your thyroid is a butterfly-shaped gland found in your neck, and it secretes hormones. It has a major role in controlling your metabolism.

If your thyroid is not functioning properly, it is possible that you have developed an overactive thyroid (hyperthyroidism), or an underactive thyroid (hypothyroidism).

If your thyroid is overactive, it makes it difficult to fall asleep, and you may also experience night sweats.

If your thyroid is underactive, then you feel sleepy and cold all the time.

Your physician can do a blood test that determines how your thyroid is functioning by measuring your levels of thyroid hormones.

Restless Legs Syndrome –

This disorder is really a neurological disorder that originates in the brain. However, it is considered a sleep disorder, as it interferes with sleep.

Symptoms include unpleasant, uncomfortable, or painful sensations in the legs that occur when inactive such as sitting or lying still. These sensations create an intense urge to move the legs, resulting in the name, "restless legs syndrome." Symptoms tend to be worse in the late afternoon and evenings, and most severe during the night when you are trying to sleep. As a result, you have difficulty falling asleep or staying asleep.

Interestingly, the symptoms can subside in the morning, which is when people affected by restless legs syndrome, can achieve their most restful sleep. In some, but not all cases, restless legs syndrome is related to another health condition, such as iron-deficiency anemia, diabetes, or peripheral neuropathy (numbness and pain that results from damage – usually due to diabetes - to nerves in your arms and legs).

Perimenopause, Menopause, and Post-Menopause –

Whether your body is just beginning to change (perimenopause), or has already gone through menopause, many women experienced disrupted sleep due to a change in hormone levels - less production of estrogen and progesterone. These sleep disruptions tend to affect the quality of sleep, not the time spent sleeping. Hot flashes, sweating, and drenched pajamas can wake women up from sleep, resulting in next-day sleepiness. Insomnia is also a common complaint of women in this stage of their lives. Hormone replacement therapy is sometimes used, or you can opt for more natural supplements such as black cohosh.

Depression –

Difficulty sleeping can be a sign of depression. Lack of sleep can also make the depression worse, as it is more difficult to cope with daily stresses when you are tired.

In addition, some people with depression sleep much more, and yet still feel fatigued all the time.

The depression can occur on its own, or it can accompany other medical issues. For example, an underactive thyroid can exhibit depression as a symptom. People with arthritis may also experience depression related to the pain that negatively affects their daily functioning.

Anxiety –

Just as with depression, anxiety can cause difficulty sleeping, or lack of sleep can cause anxiety. People with ongoing insomnia are at increased risk of developing a diagnosed anxiety disorder.

Health Consequence of Poor Sleep

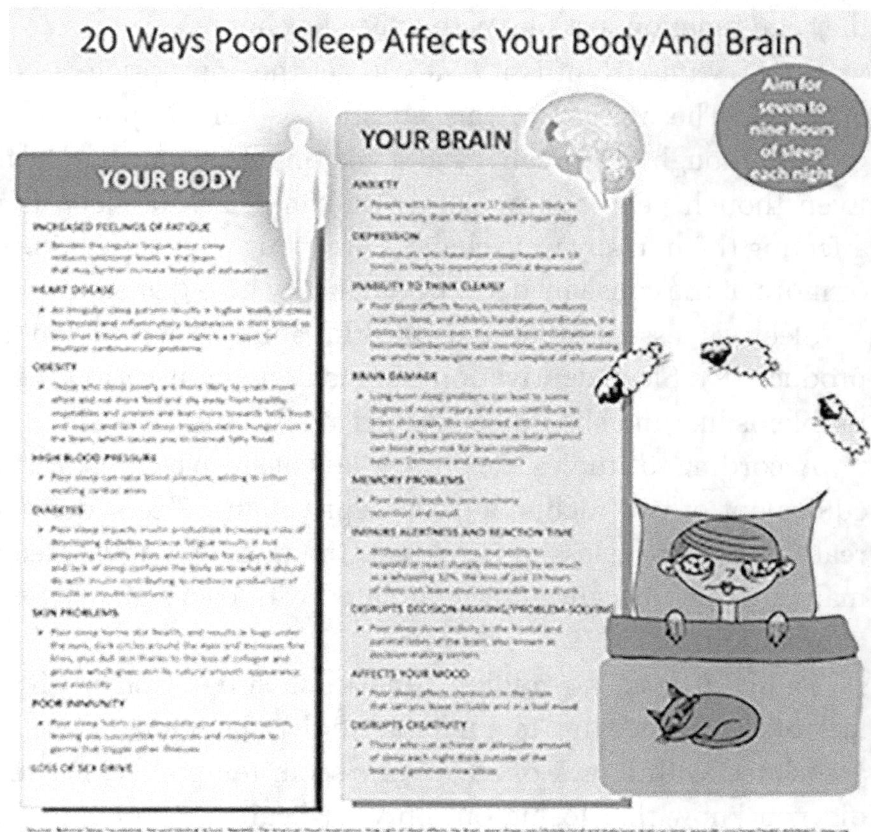

At one time or another in our lives, we've all experienced the frustration associated with a poor night's sleep. The restless nights when counting sheep become as endless as counting stars. Likely, the next day was met with numerous cups of coffee and yawns. Imagine experiencing that zombie-like feeling daily. Surely, you would tremble at the thought.

Most people would probably agree that it is necessary for everyone to get a full night's rest, while others will tell you that they can function just fine with only a few hours.

So, how important is it that you get the appropriate amount of sleep? The answer to this question is very important. Not getting enough sleep can have a major effect on your health. Even though people may feel as though a lack of sleep is not affecting them in any way, chances are, you are experiencing one or more of the consequences, whether they be big or small.

Sleep is essential to our health, ability to function and productivity. Sleep deprivation can result in many serious health problems like and should be avoided at all costs.

According to studies, 6 hours or less of sleep can result in the equivalent of two nights of sleep deprivation. Sleep "debt" is a real thing and the less of it you get; the more you must sleep to make up for it because it accumulated with every night of sleep deprivation.

Sadly, at least 50 million Americans suffer from a chronic lack of sleep according to a notable study. The immediate effects associated with a lack of sleep may seem temporary. However, did you know that losing out on your beauty rest could be the underlying cause of critical issues?

Let's consider the serious health consequences associated with a lack of sleep.

20 Health Consequences of Poor Sleep

Brain And Emotional Functioning

Anxiety and Stress

Anxiety is a common consequence of poor sleep, The National Sleep foundation reports that researchers have discovered that people with insomnia are 17 times as likely to have anxiety than those who can achieve the recommended hours of sleep. Of course, anxiety means more stress, and not getting adequate rests is hardly conducive to making sound plans in managing stress in general.

Depression

The National Sleep Foundation says that individuals who have poor sleep health are 10 times as likely to experience clinical depression. Sadly, the more often you experience insomnia, the higher your risk of developing depression.

Impaired Focus and Cognition

It is estimated that about 40 U.S. dollars are lost annually due to a lack of productivity at work. Could this be attributed to the 50 million or so Americans functioning off little sleep? When you are tired and groggy, you are unable to perform at your optimal level.

This leads to an impaired judgment which directly hinders your ability to make sound decisions. In fact, countless car accidents are a result of people falling asleep at the wheel or simply driving carelessly.

According to Mayo Clinic, simulation tests demonstrate that sleep-deprived people perform hand-eye coordination tasks as badly as or worse than intoxicated people. However, it doesn't stop there. People with poor sleep quality have an increased inability to concentrate, and zero capacity to form or retain memories.

Weakens Memory

To adequately take in information and store it for future use, you must be able to focus. As we learned previously, sleep deprivation directly influences our ability to focus. When this occurs, we are unable to process new information nor store it for future use. We may notice small changes in our memory such as forgetting deadlines, names, and even important events.

Brain Damage

Although you might think your decision to forgo sleep will only create temporary problems, Swedish researchers found that long-term sleep problems can lead to some degree of neural injury and even contribute to brain shrinkage.

According to Shape Magazine, this adverse effect combined with the increase in the levels of a toxic protein known as beta-amyloid can boost your risk for brain conditions such as Dementia and Alzheimer's.

Poor Moods

We all know how a child reacts when they miss their afternoon nap. As adults, our system reacts in a similar way when we lose sleep. Mentally, we are exhausted which leads to irritation, outbursts of anger and even depression. Our will to accomplish our tasks is reduced which may lead to feelings of tension, anxiety, and worthlessness. We may also be prone to showing aggression to others due to our agitated state.

Impairs Alertness and Reaction Time

WebMD reports that without adequate sleep, our ability to respond or react sharply decreases by as much as 32%. It's no wonder that so many accidents occur because of fatigue. According to Sleep.org, the loss of just 19 hours of sleep can leave your comparable to a drunk.

Decision Making and Problem-Solving

The ability to make firm, and well-thought-out decisions is limited because of poor sleep habits. Studies show that the frontal and parietal lobes of your brain, also known as decision-making centers, slow in activity.

Physical

Stress

When you're experiencing excessive sleep loss, your body is under a great deal of stress, which means your body is flooded with the stress hormone Cortisol. In a chronic state of stress, cortisol never leaves your body and this along with other harmful stress hormones causes a constant state of arousal that causes inflammation and has numerous detrimental effects on the mind and body. The truth is stress kills and regular healthy sleep is one of the key steps in an effective stress management plan.

Cardiovascular Disease

Lack of sleep could lead to a host of heart-related issues. The National Sleep Foundation reports that individuals who experience less sleep experience issues with glucose metabolism and blood pressure. These disruptions within the body, when left untreated, could eventually lead to heart failure, heart attacks, and strokes. The American Heart Association cites an irregular sleep pattern as being the trigger for multiple cardiovascular problems.

High Blood Pressure

Poor sleep may raise blood pressure, adding to other existing cardiac woes. If you are experiencing blood pressure problems and sleep issues, you may want to seek the attention of a sleep specialist to rule out sleep apnea.

Type 2 Diabetes

Our bodies react to sleep loss in a myriad of ways, but nothing is perhaps more amazing than the poor impact sleep can have on insulin production. WebMD reports that poor sleep can increase your risk of developing diabetes. The reason for the enhanced risk has everything to do with what it is we are putting into our bodies.

When we are tired or too fatigued to prepare healthy meals, it is in our very nature to gravitate towards those foods that can cause our sugar levels to rise rapidly. It's not all about what we eat, but our bodies response. Sleep.org reports that when we don't sleep, our body isn't always clear about what it should be doing with the insulin. This confusion contributes to a reduced production of insulin or insulin resistance.

Skin Damage

Do you ever notice how those dark circles suddenly appear under your eyes after a terrible night's sleep? Constant lack of sleep could be the blame for those and unhealthy skin. Much like your inner organs, your skin needs time to rest and recuperate. Also, since lack of sleep increases stress, the stress hormone cortisol is like a suction cup for skin elasticity. It slows down the creation of collagen thus creating lines, dark spots, and acne. They don't call it "beauty rest" for nothing.

Leads to Obesity

Author and wellness expert Dr. Michael Breus explains how our body reacts when surviving off little sleep. "Ghrelin is the 'go' hormone that tells you when to eat, and when you are sleep-deprived, you have more ghrelin." This encourages binge and mindless eating to fulfill that need. You are also less likely to go to the gym or eat nourishing foods due to your lack of energy. As this pattern persists, weight gain is inevitable.

According to the Harvard Medical School, when you don't sleep enough, you are also more likely to shy away from healthy vegetables and protein and lean more towards fatty foods and sugar. Couple this with feelings of fatigue and the desire to exercise flies out of the window.

Poor Hand and Eye Coordination

Sleep deprivation can affect primary motor skills functions, making some events awkward in execution, so if you are sleep deprived it's best to avoid activities that require hand and eye coordination.

Weakened Immune System

Loss of sleep decreases our ability to fight off sickness. As mentioned, your body never can rejuvenate itself therefore, your immune system is going on "overdrive" in a sense. Eventually, you will become more susceptible to colds, sicknesses, and bacteria. It will become much harder for your body to defend itself against these viruses.

Addiction Risks

When losing sleep becomes a habit, many people turn to sleeping aids to help them sleep through the night. Although usage of sleeping pills, when prescribed by a doctor is necessary for some, these medications are highly addictive. The sedative feeling accompanied by an already vulnerable brain can be a recipe for disaster.

Excessive Alcohol Usage

Lack of sleep can have serious consequences that affect our mood. This can increase your chance of developing depression. Unfortunately, because of these depressive symptoms, many rely on alcohol to cope. In addition, alcohol can have sedative effects that make falling asleep easier. When every night you're relying on a glass of wine to help you sleep, there may be a dependency problem brewing.

Increased Headaches

Poor sleeping habits could be the reason behind the chronic head pain. Research conducted by Dr. Paul Durham at Missouri State University found direct correlations between sleep deprivation and migraines.

He explains, " In stressful situations such as sleep deprivation, these arousal proteins occur at levels that are high enough to trigger pain."

Essentially, our body produces a series of hormones that either raise or lower our pain triggers depending on the amount of sleep we receive. Many who experience chronic sleep loss, report having frequent migraines with great intensity.

Affects Your Sex Drive

Men and women may experience lower libidos or a lack of interest in sex according to sleep specialists. This side effect is mainly due in part to inadequate energy levels, feeling tired, and higher levels of tension.

Reduced Life Quality

Considering the many ways that poor sleep affects the body, mind and spirit it is evident that continuous sleep deprivation will affect your quality of life, making it more difficult to function, be productive and be well.

Natural and Herbal Remedies for Insomnia

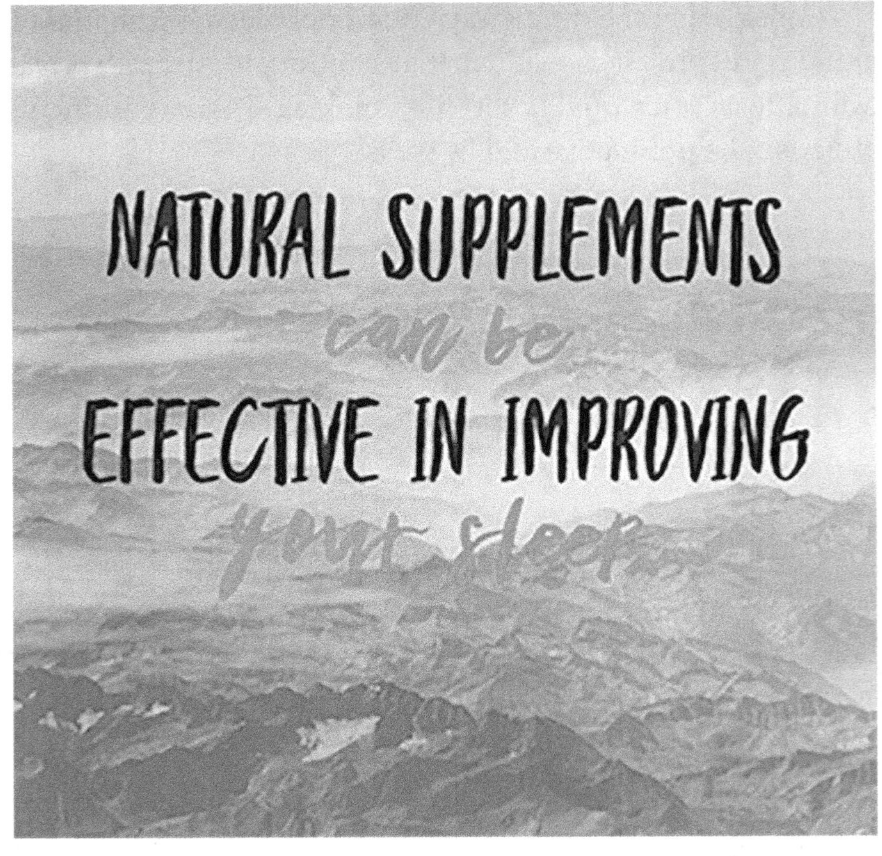

Sleep is the "secret" to functioning better at work and play and enjoying an improvement performance. According to the National Sleep Foundation people who enjoy a good night's sleep of seven hours enjoy an improved quality of life.

Regardless, you should be aiming for seven hours of sleep every night. Here are some ways to make sure that happens.

Magnesium & Calcium

These are particularly effective methods of boosting your sleep, especially when they are taken together. The bonus, of course, is that the magnesium cancels out any issues with your heart that may be caused by an increase in calcium. 600mg of calcium and 200mg of magnesium should be sufficient. Note: if you're experience diarrhea, reduce the magnesium intake.

Wild Lettuce

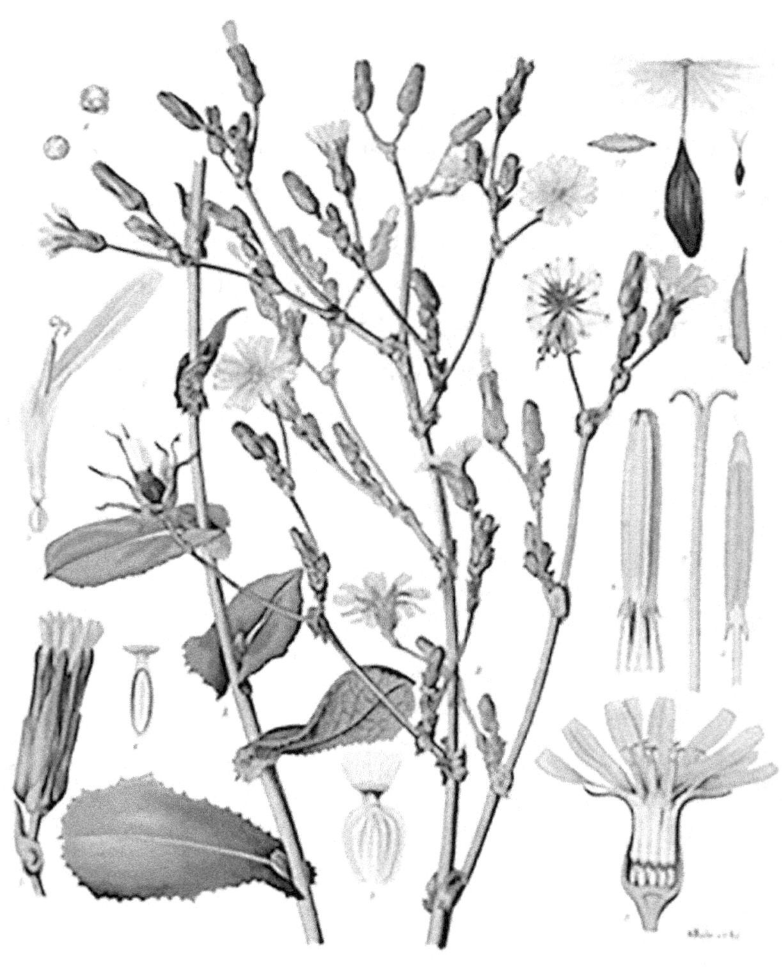

Anyone who has been dealing with headaches, muscle paint, joint pain, or anxiety may be familiar with this old trick. Wild lettuce (Lactuca virosa) is a mild sedative that is effective for occasional restlessness and both acute and chronic insomnia. It is safe for kids.

It's effective at reducing anxiety and restlessness and has even been known to help with restless leg syndrome.

Dose: Use in tincture form with 2 to 3 drops three to four times per day. If you use a supplement, take 30mg before bed. You can increase this up to 120mg if the lower isn't sufficient.

Hops

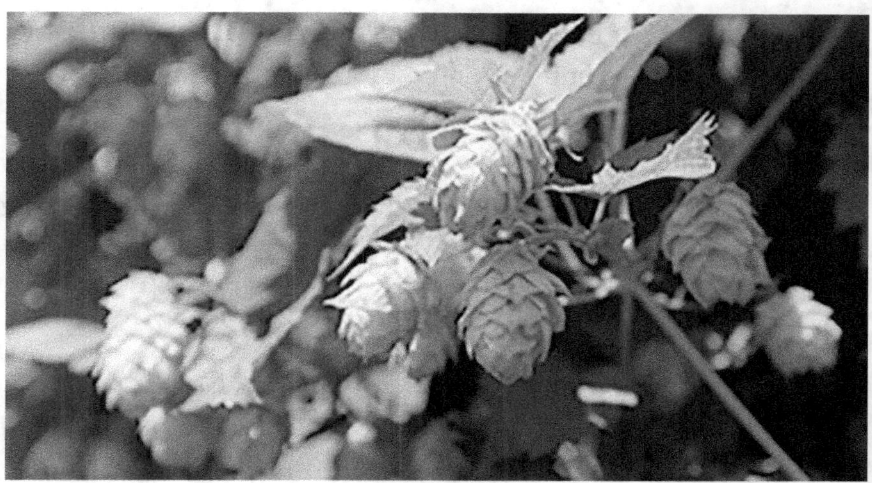

You may know this ingredient from beer, but the female flower is known for its calming effects. Hops are often additives in natural sleep aids because it is known to promote a relaxed state of mind, which is perfect for a good night's sleep. Hops also have a long history of use for nervousness, restlessness, and sleeplessness.

Dose: You can use it in a tea or in capsule form. It takes about 2 tablespoons of hops to four cups of boiling water to make a tea that you can refrigerate and reheat every night. You can also make a sachet of hops and use it as aromatherapy next to where you sleep.

Start with a dose of 30mg and work your way up to 120mg if that isn't sufficient.

Aromatherapy

This is known for its calming effects, in particular lavender. Find an oil or spray that contains real lavender and put it on your pillow every night. Alternatively, you could purchase a pillow that is lavender filled. Either way, this is a non-toxic and inexpensive way to get yourself a better night's sleep.

Melatonin

This hormone is what is controlling your sleep, so it should be no surprise that it can help induce it too. A low dose is highly effective, and high doses may increase the risk of infertility and depression.

Yoga

Meditation and yoga are an excellent way to relax before bed. There's no need to indulge in a vigorous session of yoga, as this will only serve to energize you. Rather, spend 10 minutes running through some simple and gentle yoga stretched. Additionally, 10 minutes of meditation is a great way to prepare yourself for bed. Simply spend your time focused on your breathing and shut everything else out.

L-theanine

This is the amino acid found in green tea. During the day, it provides you with a calm alertness, and in the evening, it provides you with a deeper sleep. Unfortunately, green tea isn't a sufficient source of L-theanine, not to improve your sleep. It may also increase the likelihood of night-time trips to the bathroom. There are pure supplements available, and anywhere from 50mg, right up to 200mg should be more than sufficient.

Valerian

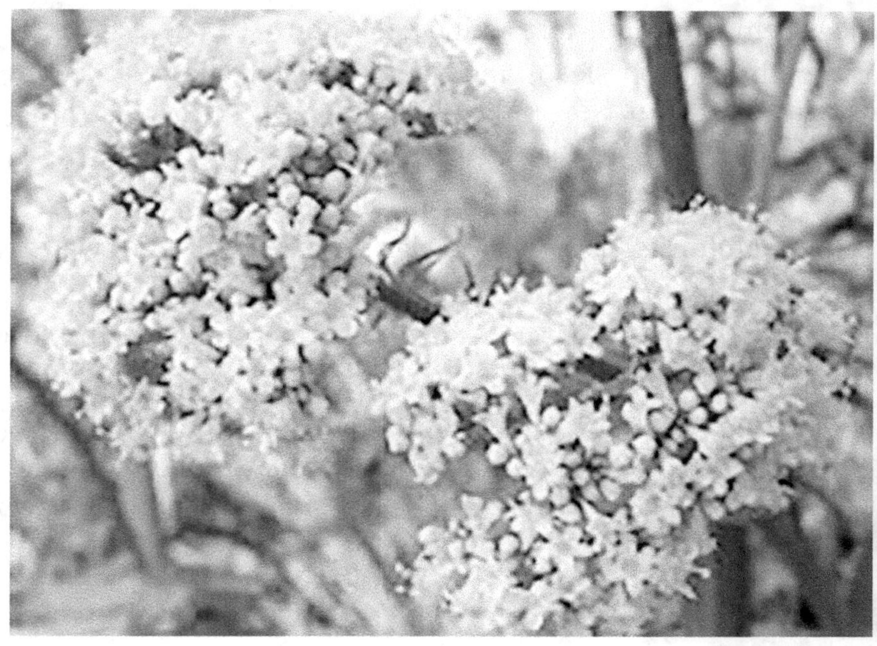

This herbal remedy is commonly used in Europe, where herbal remedies are most popular. Valerian (Valeriana officinalis) increases the amount of the neurochemical GABA, which stands for gamma aminobutyric acid. This neurotransmitter, when released, reduces anxiety and makes it easier to sleep. Valerian is a great option for those who have a hard time falling asleep and it reduces nighttime waking. Valerian is an all-natural herbal sedative that does not have any of the dangerous side effects or addictive properties of Valium and other prescription sedatives under the benzodiazepine category. It also works well in combination with other sedative herbs, including, skullcap, California poppy, hops, and passionflower.

This is perhaps insomniacs most preferred and common sleep remedies to turn to. It increases the speed of falling asleep, the cycle of deep sleep, and your overall quality of sleep, too. Valerian is most effective when it is used over an extended period.

Dose: It can be taken in capsule, tincture or tea form. One teaspoon of dried valerian root can be mixed with hot water and steeped for around fifteen minutes to release its active ingredients and drank as needed. For tincture use 2 to 5 drops two to three times per day.

200mg should be sufficient, though you can take as much as 800mg. Do note, though, that for around 10% of people it will have the opposite effect. If you find valerian makes you energized, take it during the day.

Chamomile

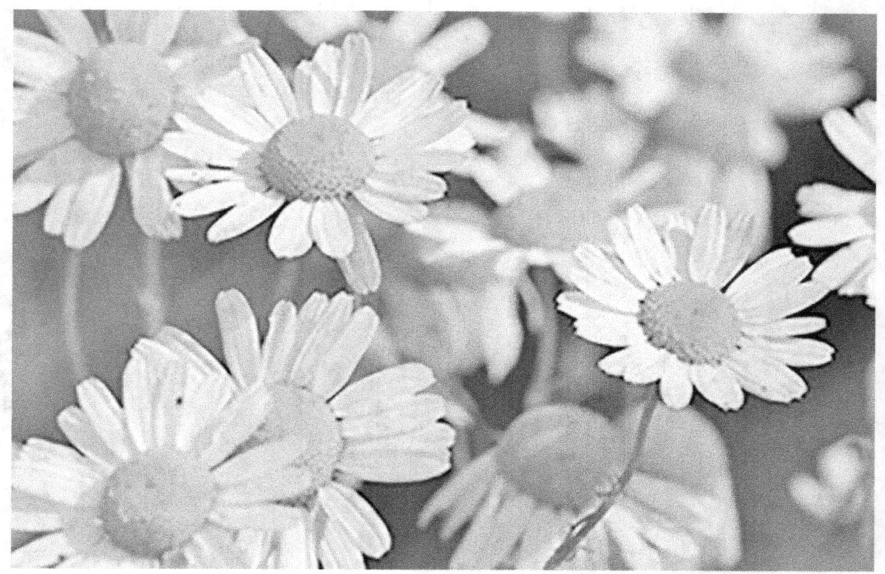

This is a popular sleep aid, usually taken in tea form. It contains a substance known as apigenin, which mimics GABA in the brain. By turning on GABA receptors, it induces a state of relaxation and helps you feel tired enough to sleep.

Dose: Take two tablespoons of dry chamomile flowers and brew it with hot water. Lemon juice, milk, and/or honey can be used to spice up and flavor the tea, although it tastes great on its own.

Cherry Juice

Alcohol will only serve to disrupt your sleep cycle, so if you're intent on having a nightcap, make it this one. Cherry juice just happens to be high in melatonin. So, opt for a small glass of tart cherry juice half an hour before bed.

Lavender

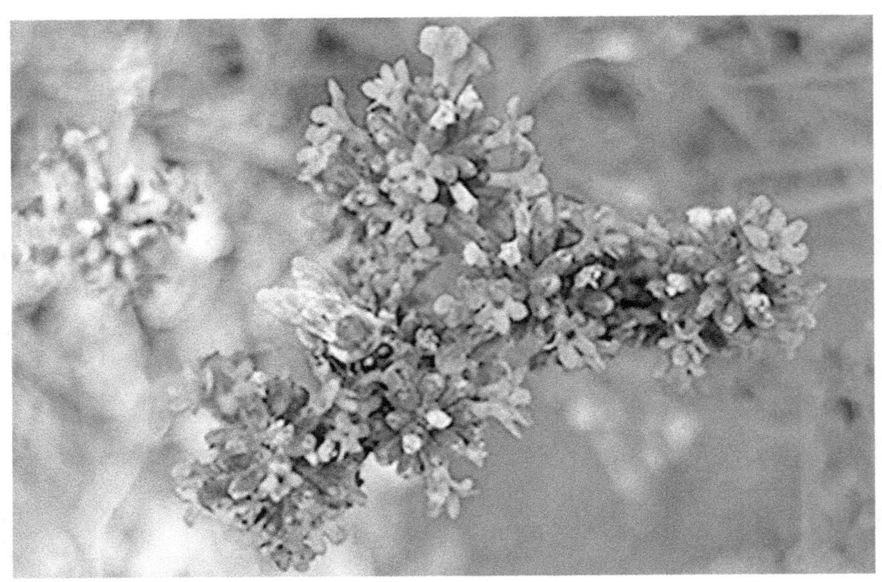

Lavender (Lavandula angustifolia) is good as an aromatherapy remedy for the induction of sleep and has no side effects. Lavender has been shown in research studies to bring on brain wave patterns like sleep.

A study conducted at Britain's University of Southampton tracked sleep patterns of 10 adults. For one week, 5 of the adults slept in a room where the air was diffused with lavender essential oil, while the other 5 participants slept in a room diffused with a placebo (sweet almond oil). For the second week, the participants switched rooms. The results of the study showed that participants ranked their sleep quality as being 20% better on average in the lavender-scented room versus the one scented with placebo.

Another study conducted by psychologists at Wesleyan University found that 31 men and women who sniffed lavender essential oil versus distilled water for only four 2-minute periods before bedtime slept more soundly as shown by their sleep cycles and brain scans. Moreover, the participants who smelled lavender reported sleeping more soundly and feeling more energetic the next morning.

Dose: You don't eat Lavender but use it as aromatherapy, either in a diffuser or in a sachet next to your pillow. There are also essential oil candles, and essential oil drops can be added to a hot bath for relaxation before bedtime. Be sure to use only high quality essential oils for best results.

Passion Flower

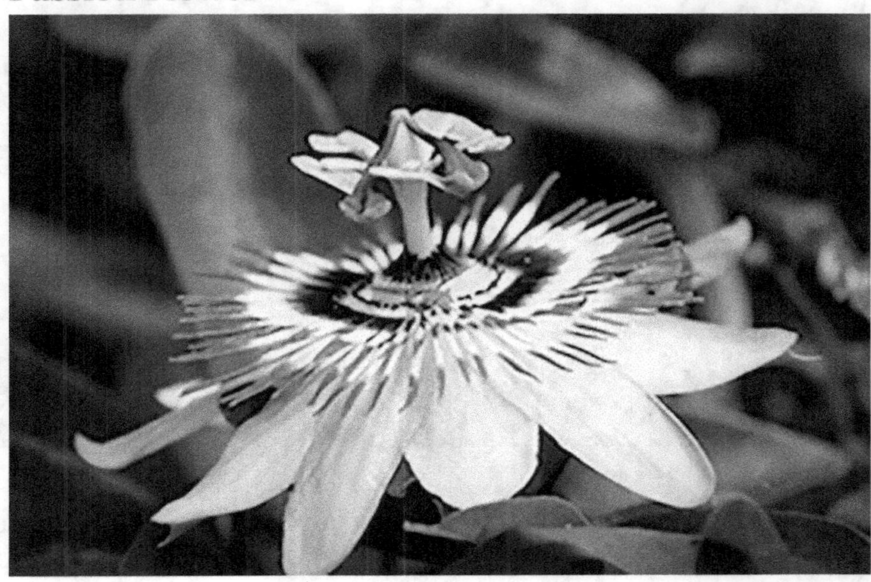

Passion flower (Passiflora incarnata) is an effective herb for use in insomnia that is caused by mental worry, overwork, or nervous exhaustion. It is a common ingredient in forty different sedative preparations sold in England. Herbalists advocate its use for both kids and adults as it has no side effects even when used in large doses.

Dose: Passion flower can be drank in tea form or used as a tincture with 30 to 60 drops taken 3 to 4 times per day.

California Poppy

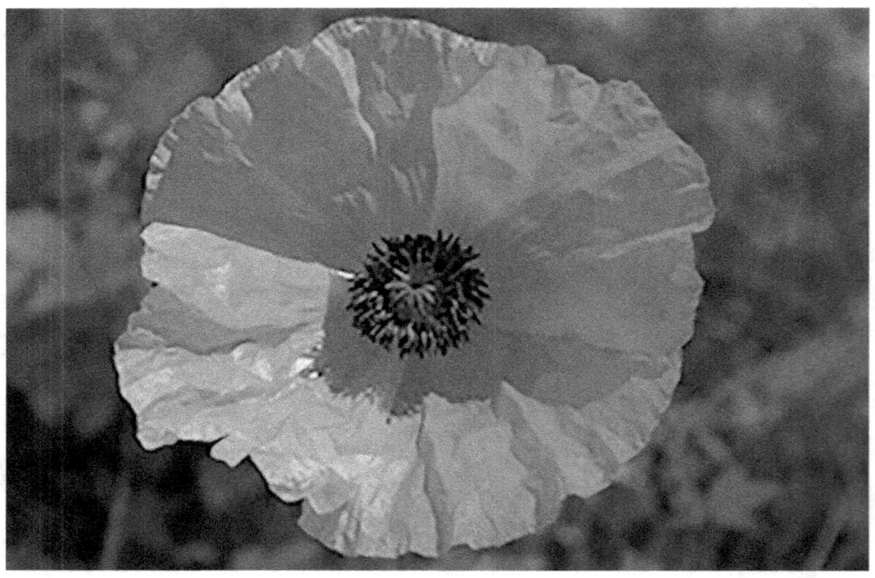

California poppy (Eschscholzia californica) is a wonderful natural treatment for insomnia; it induces relaxation and eases mild anxiety. It is mild enough for use in children.

Studies have shown California poppy to be an effective plant sedative with anti-anxiety properties. One study conducted in 1995 showed it to improve both quality and latency of sleep.

Dose: California poppy can be taken in tea form or as a tincture (a much stronger form than the tea) with 30 to 40 drops two to three times per day.

Kava Kava

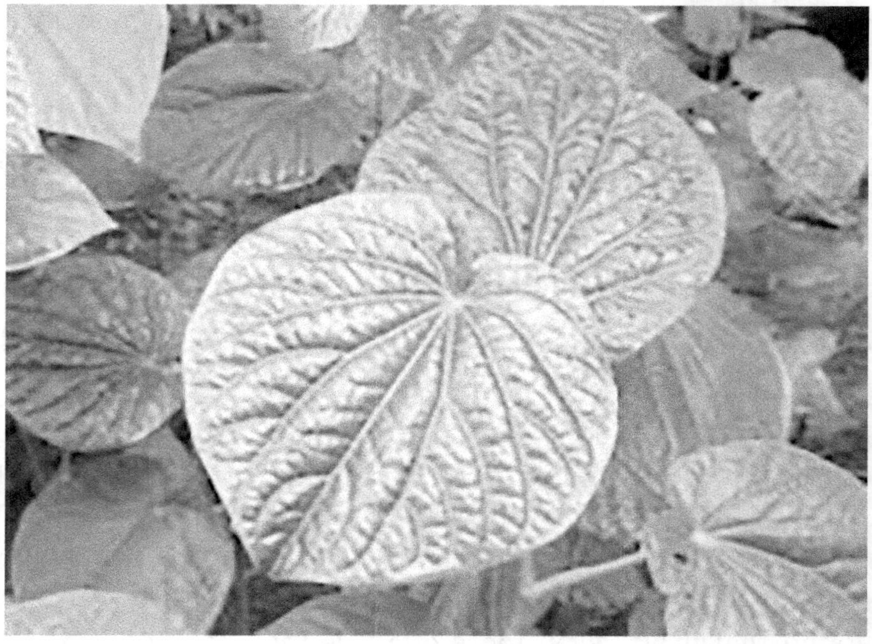

Kava kava (Piper methysticum) is often used for it relaxation benefits. It's all-natural sedative effect is ideal for insomnia, acute sleeplessness and fatigue.

Dose: Drink 1 cup of Kava Kava tea two to three times per day. It can also be used as a tincture with 3 to 4 drops two to three times per day.

Milk & Honey

This is another excellent nightcap option. Milk contains tryptophan, you know, that magical amino acid in turkey that makes everyone nap after Thanksgiving dinner? By enjoying a glass of warm milk before bed, you'll increase your serotonin levels, thus triggering this sedative. Honey is a carb and will help the hormone transmit to your brain quicker.

Turkey

Now, you *should* avoid eating before bed because it can lead to heartburn. However, if you *are* feeling hungry there are a few foods that can help. A turkey sandwich delivers tryptophan and carbs just like milk and honey does. So, will a banana and milk. If you're truly hungry and know, you won't be able to sleep over the sounds of your stomach growling, make a smart decision.

Cognitive Behavioral Therapy

CBT tends to be focused on finding out what thoughts are triggering stress and depression. However, it may be the best natural remedy to deal with insomnia. It may be able to help you retain your body for a faster and deeper sleep. A Harvard Study found that it was even more effective than prescribed sleeping pills. Participants not only saw an improvement in the quality of their sleep, but also in the speed of falling asleep. The National Sleep Foundation suggests that you keep a sleep diary. Note down when you go to bed, as well as when you wake up. Forget taking naps during the day and follow a regular sleep schedule.

Always get up at the same time and always go to bed at the same time.

Herbal Tea

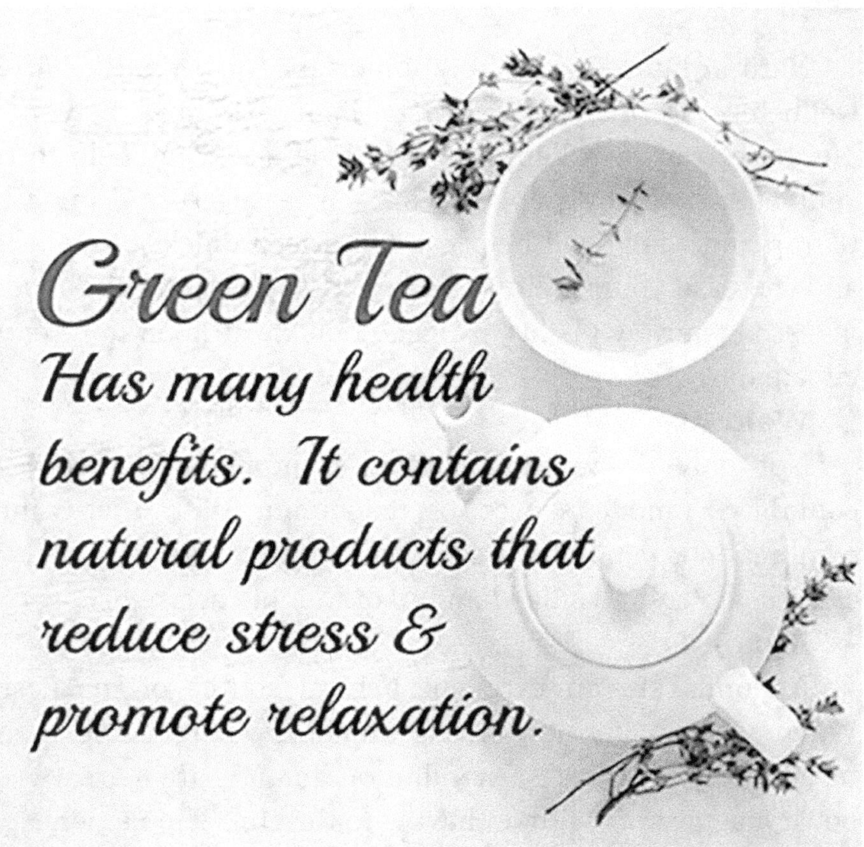

Whether you choose valerian tea or chamomile tea, herbal teas are an effective remedy to handle insomnia. You can find these teas anywhere and you should enjoy them around 30 minutes before bed. Another effective herbal tea is passionflower tea.

A Hot Bath

Women who suffer from insomnia have been found to have a much better time of getting to sleep if they enjoy a hot bath. Ideally, aim for ninety minutes of soaking in a hot tub.

Light Therapy

Natural light is incredibly important for overall health and wellbeing. Dermatologists offer light therapy, or you can purchase your own light box for home use. They help to reset your body clock by shipping your sleep patterns. Using a light therapy box daily will help you fall asleep quicker, stay asleep, and increase your quality of sleep. If you're not quite ready to invest in your own light box, head outside at noon to reset your circadian rhythm.

Walnuts

Not only do walnuts contain tryptophan, but they also contain a unique source of melatonin. With that winning combination, you'll soon see that it won't take long to get to sleep if you enjoy a small handful of walnuts before bed.

Almonds

Almonds are an excellent natural source of magnesium. When your magnesium levels are low, you're going to have trouble staying asleep. A handful of almonds are a great way to boost magnesium, without having to turn to a supplement.

Dairy

It isn't just warm milk that helps you get off to sleep, any dairy product will do. While cheese may not be the go to, yogurt is effective.

Side Salad

Enjoying a leafy green salad at dinner time may just help you sleep later. This is because lettuce contains lactucarium, this works as a sedative and affects your brain as opium would. You can also create a lettuce tea to enjoy before bed. Simmer three large lettuce leaves in a cup of hot water for around 15 minutes. Add a couple of sprigs of mint after you remove it from the heat and sip on it around half an hour before bed.

Tortilla Chips & Pretzels

These food items have high on the glycemic index, causing a spike in insulin and blood sugar. In turn, this will shorten the time it will take for you to fall asleep. Normally you'd want these to stay level to avoid other problems; however, if you need rest, this is a great way to induce sleep.

Cereal

Enjoying a bowl of carbohydrate rich cereal is an excellent way to get yourself off to sleep. It combined calcium, tryptophan, and carbs for the ultimate sleep-inducing combination.

Chickpeas

Chickpeas are another excellent source of tryptophan. A light snack before bed may not be a terrible idea if it's hummus with a few whole grain crackers.

St John's Wort

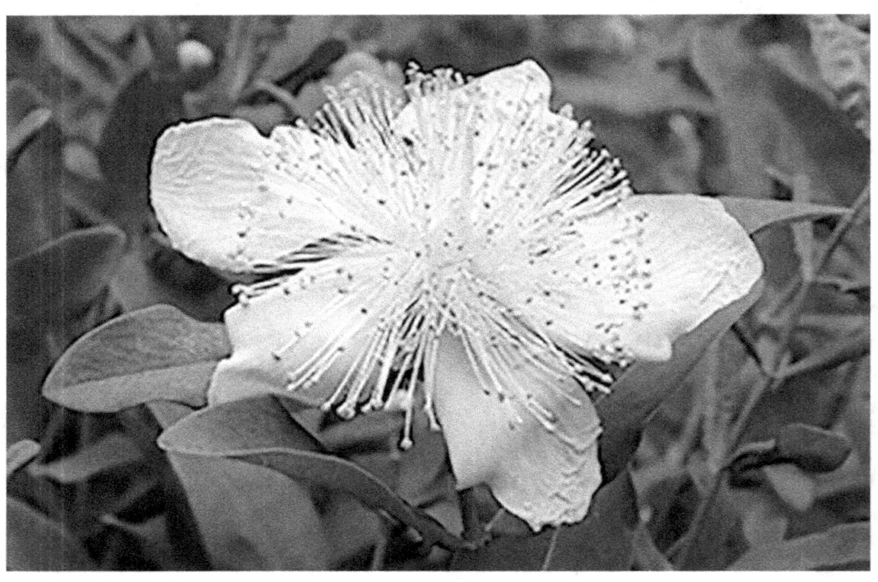

This is often used to reduce the symptoms of depression. This may just be exactly what you need to help with your sleep problem, and depression is a common cause of insomnia.

St. John's Wort (Hypericum perforatum) is a common anti-depressant in Europe and dates to ancient Greece. It is being discovered in the US as a great way of raising serotonin levels in the brain and improving sleep. When there is more serotonin, the sleep-inducing melatonin increases as well so that you can get a restful night's sleep. Modern scientific studies have shown St. John's Wort to help with chronic insomnia and to alleviate certain types of mild depression. It mixes well with lemon balm for an additive effect.

Dose: You can take 2 teaspoons of the dried herbal tops and flowers of the St. John's Wort plant and steep it for 5-10 minutes to make a tea or you can take a prepared capsule. For tincture, use 1/2 to 1 teaspoon two to three times per day. It typically takes about 2-3 weeks for the full therapeutic effect to take place. St. John's Work causes sensitivity to light, so exposure to sun while taking it is not recommended. Should you experience light sensitivity or any unpleasant symptoms, stop use, and consult with a qualified herbalist.

Screens Off

We live in a technological world, and unfortunately, this often creates a dependency that keeps us up at night. Turn the TV off, put your phone and tablet down, and spend the hour before bedtime living like a luddite. Go for a bath, read a book, or spend this time doing yoga or in meditation.

Exercise

Regular exercise is a great way to ensure that you're getting a good night's sleep. You'll have more energy for your waking hours and enjoy a restful sleep at night. You should never exercise just before bed, though, as you'll end up wide awake.

Lemon Balm

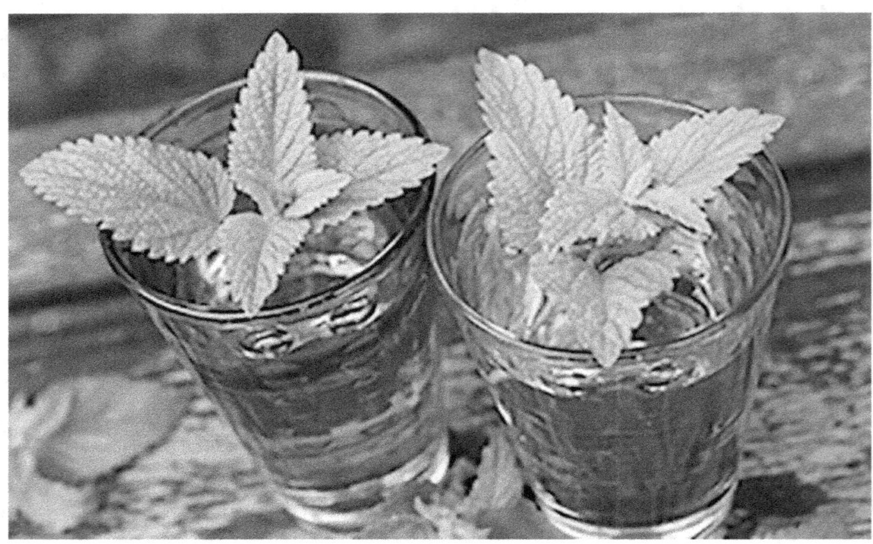

Lemon balm is a commonly used herb in Traditional Chinese Medicine. It has many uses, one of which is to raise serotonin levels, which promotes sleep.

This ancient herb's been used for thousands of years. Once upon a time, it was considered a cure all, treating snake bites, and asthma. Now, however, it's used for promoting relaxation and calmness, as well as to lift mood. Depression is linked to sleeplessness, so lemon balm is an effective way to get sleep, as it will promote mental health. It brags sedative effects; however, a high dosage can create anxiety. Create your own lemon balm tea. If you're using fresh lemon balm, you'll need eight tablespoons, and for the dried stuff two tablespoons. Add two teaspoons of chamomile, and honey to taste.

Dose: Make a tea using 8-10 tablespoons of fresh lemon balm (about 2 tablespoons when dried) and mix it with a couple of teaspoons of dried chamomile flowers then steep with water. It takes about forty-five minutes to work so schedule your tea drinking accordingly.

Noise

While some people may need total silence to get sleep, this is untrue for others. Your brain is still processing noise, even while you're asleep, so certain noises can increase anxiety, the faucet dripping, a clock ticking, even the electricity humming. If something jars you awake in the middle of the night, it isn't the noise itself, it's the inconsistency in what you're hearing. You can beat this by using white noise. It's soothing, and it fills the silence. It can be as simple as turning a fan on, however, there are apps for it or you can purchase a sound machine.

Catnip

It may send cats round the bend, but for you... it has a sedative effect. Add two teaspoons of dried catnip to eight ounces of boiling water and drizzle honey to taste. If you're using fresh catnip, you will need four teaspoons. Drink it half an hour before bed.

Pajamas

Whether you prefer to sleep in flannel character pajamas, boxers, or your birthday suit always, have a specific outfit for your bedtime. This will signal your body and brain that it's time for sleep.

Give Up

If you've been in bed for half an hour and you're still unable to sleep, just give up. Get up and read a book until you start to feel tired, and then go back to bed to try it again. Sometimes the inability to sleep can just increase your anxiety and stress levels, creating an upset that will prevent you from falling asleep.

Thoughts

Before you go rushing out to the drug store to clear the shelves of the over the counter sleep medications, you should try these natural remedies and make smart decisions in your daily life.

Cut out caffeine after two in the afternoon and avoid eating right before bed. Consider creating a bedtime routine that will help relax you before sleep. Whether you prefer a spot of meditation, or a hot bath, anything that will help calm your mind is going to help you get a good night's sleep.

As tempting as it may be to have a nip of whiskey before bed, you're only preventing yourself from having a restful sleep. Poor sleep can have a serious impact on every aspect of your life, so it is vital that you take the necessary steps to get your body back on track.

Everyone reacts to herbal sleep medications differently, so it is a good idea to keep trying different formulations to find what works best for you.

Caution: Talk to your doctor about taking an herbal sleep remedy, especially if you are on other types of medication that can interfere with it. Herbs are powerful plants, and some are contraindicated with certain medications.

It is always a good idea to consult with an herbalist, who is a specialist in herbal remedies as they can advise you on the best herbs and doses for your insomnia condition.

The Link Between Insomnia & Anxiety in Children & Teens – What Parents Can Do to Help

Is insomnia in children and teens like adults?

Yes, children can also have insomnia. In fact, a poll done by the National Sleep Foundation found that more than two out of three children ten years old and under have had a sleep issue of some sort.

Insomnia may last for only a few days (due to sickness), or it can become more frequent and long-term. Sometimes this can be indicative of anxiety, depression, or other medical problems, so you should always make sure to have your child evaluated by a physician.

Obviously, children and teens may have different **reasons** for their insomnia when compared to adults. For example, children may fear the monsters they think exist in their closets or under their beds. Teens may be stressed by exams or bullying going on at school. In many cases, there is a component of anxiety that coexists with the insomnia. That is why it is important to try to get to the **root cause** of the insomnia whenever possible. In some cases, there is no reason for the insomnia, however.

The signs and symptoms of insomnia in children and teens can include:

- Sleepiness during the day
- Poor performance in school
- Irritability
- Anxiety
- Decreased focus and concentration
- Mood swings
- Being worried about things
- Hyperactivity
- Forgetfulness and decreased memory for things
- Increased behavioral issues such as fighting and not getting along with others
- Increased impulsiveness

Because children and teens with insomnia have been found to have increased risk for anxiety disorders and depression, it is important to recognize the signs and symptoms of insomnia in your children and teens so that you can help ensure they get the sleep they need.

Here are some ways to help a child or teen with insomnia:

- **Try to determine the cause of the insomnia first**

For example, if you learn that your child is stressed by trying to keep up with school and homework as well as out-of-school extracurricular activities, you will need to address this before the insomnia can go away. This can be quite a common stressor for children and teens, as they tend to be overscheduled.

- **Once you determine the cause, try to eliminate the stressor**

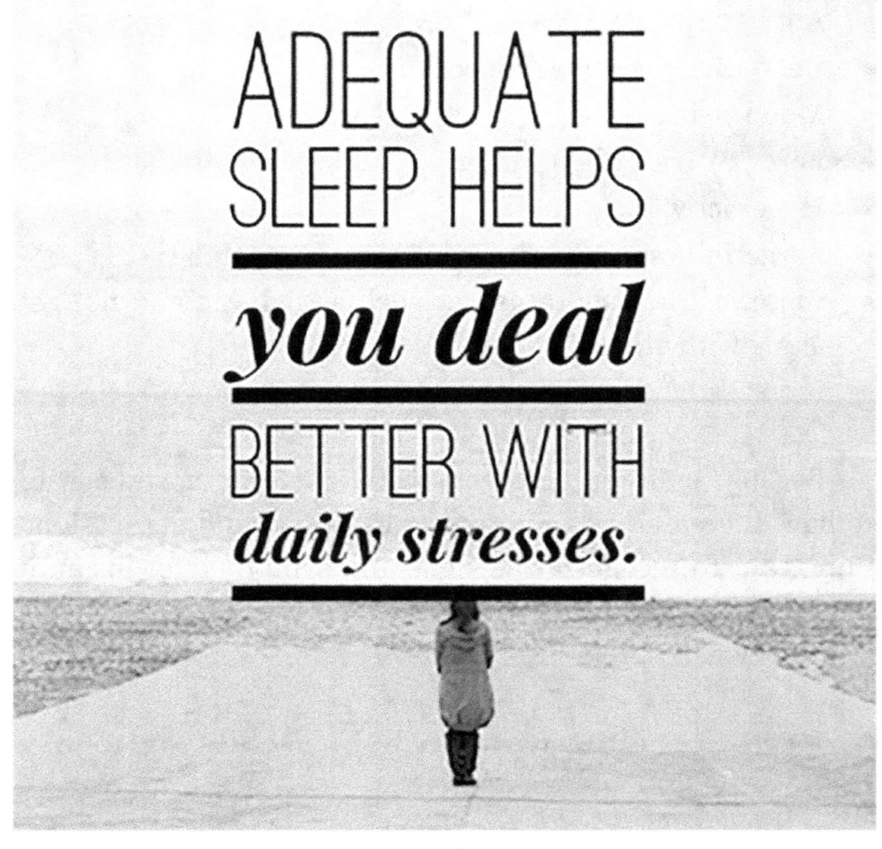

In the example above, if the problem is the child feeling stressed by an overly busy schedule, you will need to adjust the schedule. It may involve talking to the teacher and setting realistic expectations for homework. Perhaps you will learn that your child is not using his time effectively at school and home, and he therefore needs more guidance on how to do this.

Many children and teens are poor managers of their time, and they will need your help in this area. To do this, you may need to set limits on use of technology such as video games, for example. It may also be helpful to sit down and help your child determine how to prioritize tasks.

- **Establish and follow a bedtime routine**

Just like younger children do well with a set routine every night, so do older children (and even adults). It gets your mind and body prepared for sleep. When you have a set routine, it also keeps things predictable and allows you to manage your time better.

You need to teach children and teens that they need time to unwind and relax before going to sleep. This means no television, video games, social media, and so forth for one to two hours before going to bed. These bright devices can also interfere with melatonin production in your body, which helps tell your body that it is time to go to sleep.

Instead, teach them that they can do something relaxing such as reading a book before turning off the light, if they are old enough. Invest in special lightbulbs that do not emit blue light. Red lightbulbs are also an option, and you can find them online.

For younger children, you can set up a specific routine of having a bedtime snack, then teeth brushing, you read them a book, and then tuck them into bed with a hug and kiss. It may also help to provide your child with a back rub or some extra cuddling time. You just must determine what works best for your own children.

- **Limit your child's or teen's access to the news**

Unfortunately, the news media portrays a lot of violent and terrible things happening in the world – from terrorist activities to inclement weather such as tornadoes and floods. For an already-anxious child, this can severely contribute to insomnia.

- **Do not discuss anxiety-provoking or stressful situations before bedtime**

Before your child goes to bed, it is not the time to discuss your disappointment in your child's grades or that he forgot to do his chores again.

- **Teach your older child stress management and anxiety-reducing techniques**

Children with insomnia can benefit from many of the same stress and anxiety reduction techniques that adults use – progressive muscle relaxation, visual imagery, yoga, deep diaphragmatic breathing.

Learning these methods and using them before bed, can help treat insomnia as they can turn on the relaxed, parasympathetic part of your nervous system.

- **Teach and use good sleep hygiene methods**

These methods include waking up and going to bed at the same time, avoiding napping, and avoiding caffeinated beverages and foods six hours before bedtime.

Ensure the bed is only used for sleep, and that it is not the place where the child watches television or does other activities during the day.

In addition, do not exercise two hours before bedtime. However, do keep in mind that exercise is important in helping with quality sleep so do ensure you do promote exercise. The best kinds of activities can be those where you spend time with your child going for a walk, riding a bike, or going to the park.

Also teach your older child that instead of tossing and turning for too long, it is better to get out of bed, put a light on low (preferably a red lightbulb), and do something quiet such as reading for 15 minutes, and then go back to bed and attempt to sleep. If sleep does not occur soon after returning to bed, then he can get up again, and repeat the process until sleep finally does come.

- **Set up the bedroom for rest and relaxation**

This means sleeping in a room that is not overly hot. It is recommended that you keep the room between 68 and 70 degrees Fahrenheit (20 – 21 degrees Celsius). It really does depend on the age of the child and if/what types of pajamas the child wears to bed.

Have drapes in place to keep the room dark during sleeping, but you can have a small unobtrusive nightlight (with a red lightbulb) in a corner of the room, if necessary to lessen anxiety. If your child tends to stare at the alarm clock numbers, then it is best to turn it around to make sure that it is not able to be viewed.

- **Remove technology devices from the bedroom**

Remove any temptation to check the time, text messages, emails, or social media for the latest updates. This can increase anxiety, especially if there is anything unsettling that your child reads or views just before it is time to go to sleep. The blue light emitted from these devices also suppresses melatonin – the sleep hormone – production, thereby delaying sleep further.

In children with anxiety, removal of the devices during the day can also be helpful. Initially, it may cause more anxiety due to the fear of not being accessible by others and no longer "being in the loop" always. This FOMO, or Fear of Missing Out, can be anxiety provoking. However, you can teach your children that being "on call" all the time or knowing every little thing about other people's lives (through social media), can cause them more anxiety which further contributes to sleep problems.

- **Spend extra time with your children and teens**

When you spend time talking and doing fun things together (i.e. family board game night), your children and teens feel closer to you, will trust you more, and will open to you more. This gives you the opportunity to get a better idea of what they are experiencing in their lives, and how it may be contributing to their insomnia and anxiety. Many times, you can also help reduce the insomnia by helping them deal with or solve the problems they are facing. You must remember that children and teens do not have the life experience and knowledge of how to deal with situations like you do. By simply providing them with this guidance and teaching, you can help reduce the anxiety too.

In addition, you want to remember that you want to teach them methods of how they can deal with stressors when you are not there. You may want to do role playing to give them the confidence to deal with situations that arise when you cannot be present.

- **Consult a physician or naturopathic doctor**

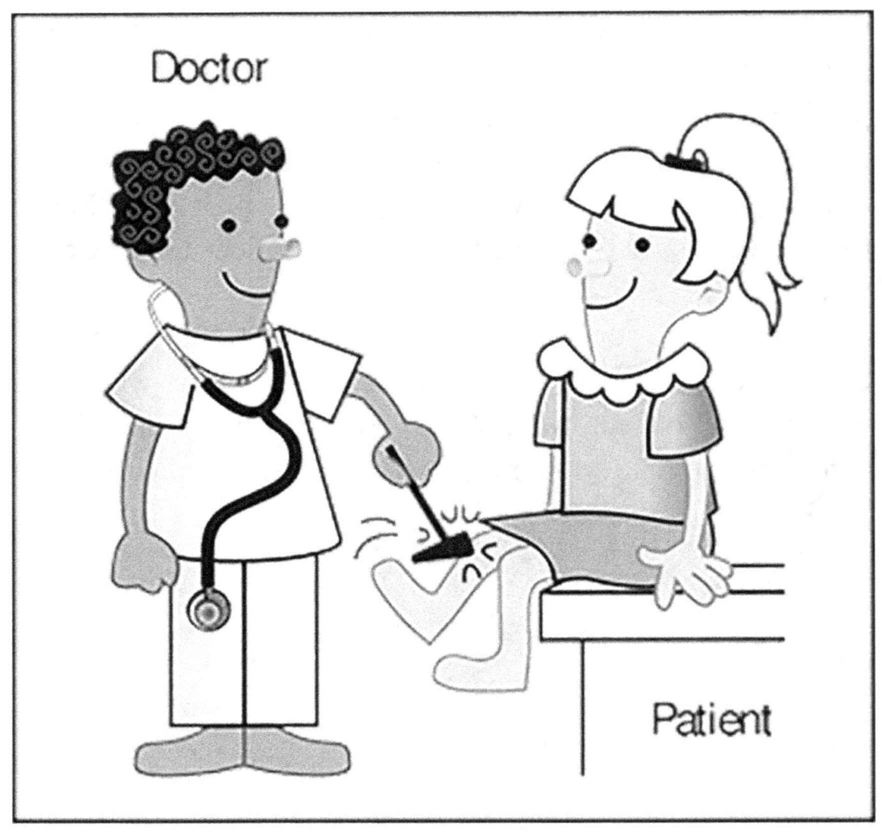

Sometimes, more help is needed. Medications are not generally prescribed for children with insomnia. However, alternative treatment options may include cognitive-behavioral therapy. The physician or pediatrician can make a referral to a therapist or psychologist trained in this.

A naturopathic doctor may also be able to provide natural suggestions for improving sleep too.

In any case, it is always important for the healthcare professional to try to determine if there is a physical or psychological cause to the insomnia.

Conclusion

Insomnia is a problem for adults, children, and teens. Anxiety often co-exists in individuals with insomnia, and it becomes important to identify the source of the anxiety if insomnia is to be treated successfully. There are many methods that can be used to help a child with insomnia, which have been outlined above.

www.ingramcontent.com/pod-product-compliance
Lightning Source LLC
Chambersburg PA
CBHW070136260726
48658CB00001B/437